The Tasty Guide to Plant-Based Dinner

Amazing Dinner Recipes to Improve Your Plant-Based Diet and Manage Your Weight

I0135328

Carl Brady

Table of contents

Butternut Squash Chipotle Chili

Preparation time: 10 minutes Cooking time: 60 minutes
Servings: 4

Ingredients:

3 cups cooked black beans 2 Avocados, pitted, peeled, diced 1 small butternut squash, peeled, ½-inch cubed 1 medium red onion, peeled, chopped 2 teaspoons minced garlic 1 tablespoon chopped chipotle pepper in adobo 14 ounces diced tomatoes with the juices 2 medium red bell peppers, chopped ¼ teaspoon ground cinnamon 1 tablespoon red chili powder 1 ½ teaspoon salt 1 teaspoon ground cumin 1 bay leaf 2 tablespoons olive oil 2 cups vegetable broth 3 corn tortillas

Directions: Cook onion, squash, and bell pepper in oil into a large stockpot placed over medium heat for 5 minutes. Switch heat to medium-low level, add peppers, garlic, cumin, cinnamon, and chili powder, stir until mixed and cook for 30 seconds. Then add remaining ingredients, except for tortilla, stir until combined and cook for 1 hour until done, adjusting the taste halfway. Meanwhile, prepare the tortilla chips and for this, cut tortillas into 2 by ¼ inch strips, place a skillet pan over medium heat, add oil and when hot, toss in tortilla strips, sprinkle with some salt and cook for 7 minutes until golden. When done, transfer tortilla chips to a plate lined with paper towels and serve with cooked chili.

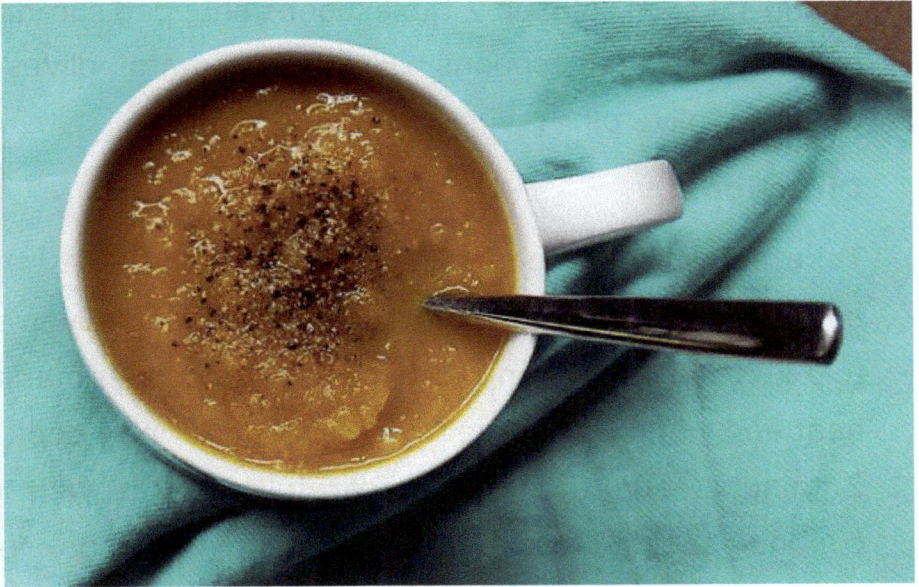

Hummus Quesadillas

Preparation time: 5 minutes Cooking time: 8 minutes Servings: 1

Ingredients:

1 tortilla, whole-grain, about 8-inches 1/3 cup hummus ¼ cup sautéed spinach 2 tablespoons chopped sun-dried tomatoes 2 tablespoons sliced Kalamata olives 1 teaspoon olive oil

Directions:

Take a tortilla, spread hummus on its one side, then cover its one-half with spinach, tomatoes, and olives and fold it. Take a medium skillet pan, place it over medium heat and when hot, place folded quesadilla in it, cook for 2 minutes and then flip it carefully. Brush with oil, continue cooking for 2 minutes, flip again and cook for 2 minutes until golden brown. When done, transfer quesadilla to a cutting board, slice it into wedges and serve

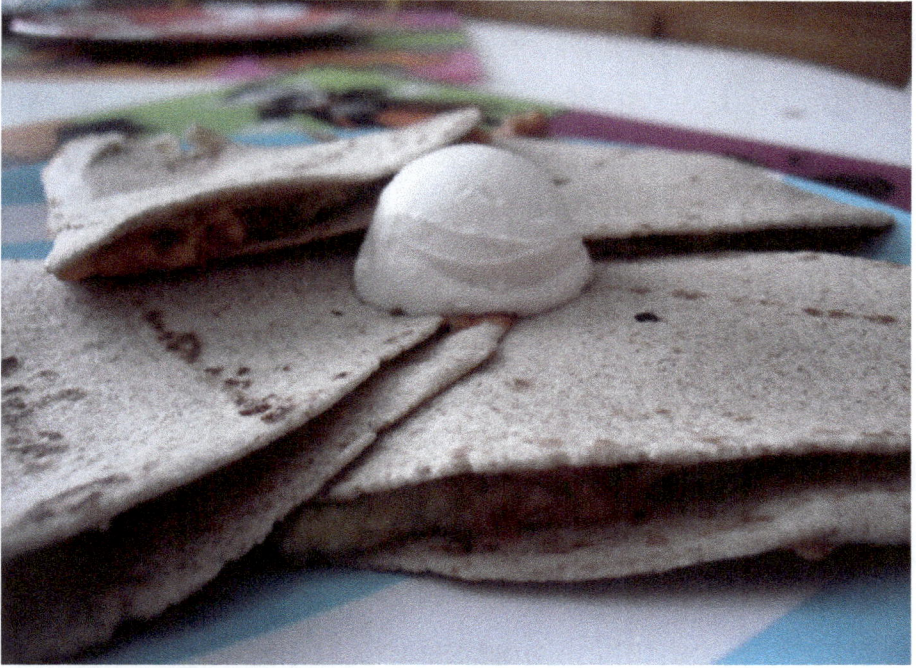

Kale Salad

Preparation time: 10 minutes Cooking time: 0 minute Servings: 4

Ingredients:

For the Salad: ½ of avocado, sliced ½ bunch of kale, chopped 2 carrots, sliced into long ribbons 1 radish, chopped ¼ cup cherry tomatoes 2 tablespoons green pumpkin seeds, toasted 1 cup cooked brown rice

For Green Tahini: 1 small jalapeño, deseeded, chopped ½ cup cilantro ½ teaspoon minced garlic ½ teaspoon ground cumin ¼ teaspoon red pepper flakes ¼ teaspoon of sea salt 1/3 cup olive oil 2 tablespoons tahini 1/3 cup lime juice 1 ½ teaspoon honey

Directions:

Prepare the tahini, and for this, place all its ingredients in a food processor and pulse for 2 minutes until blended. Then prepare the salad and for this, place all its ingredients in a bowl and toss until mixed. Add prepared tahini dressing, toss until coated, and serve.

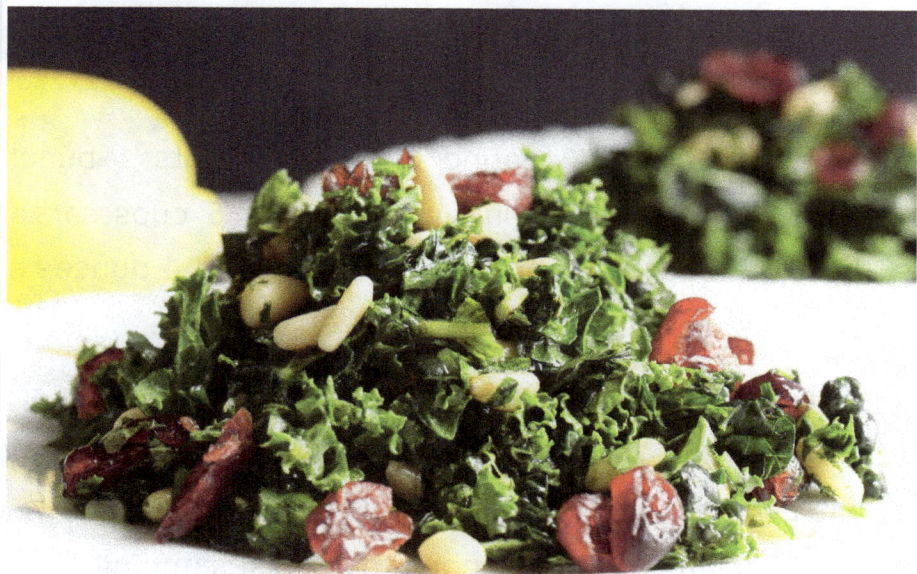

Peanut Slaw with Soba Noodles

Preparation time: 40 minutes Cooking time: 0 minute Servings: 4

Ingredients:

For the Slaw: ½ pound Brussels sprouts 1 bunch of green onions, sliced into thin rounds 6 cups shredded green cabbage 4 medium carrots, grated 4 ounces soba noodles, cooked

For the Peanut Dressing: 1 teaspoon minced garlic 1 tablespoon grated ginger 2 tablespoons honey 3 tablespoons rice vinegar 3 tablespoons soy sauce ½ cup peanut butter 3 tablespoons toasted sesame oil

For the Garnish: ¼ cup chopped cilantro 2 tablespoons chopped peanuts 1 lime, sliced into wedges

Directions:

Prepare the dressing and for this, place all its ingredients in a large bowl and whisk until smooth. Place noodles in a large bowl, add all the vegetables, pour in the prepared dressing and toss until well coated. Let the slaw marinate for 30 minutes, top with peanuts and cilantro and serve with lime wedges

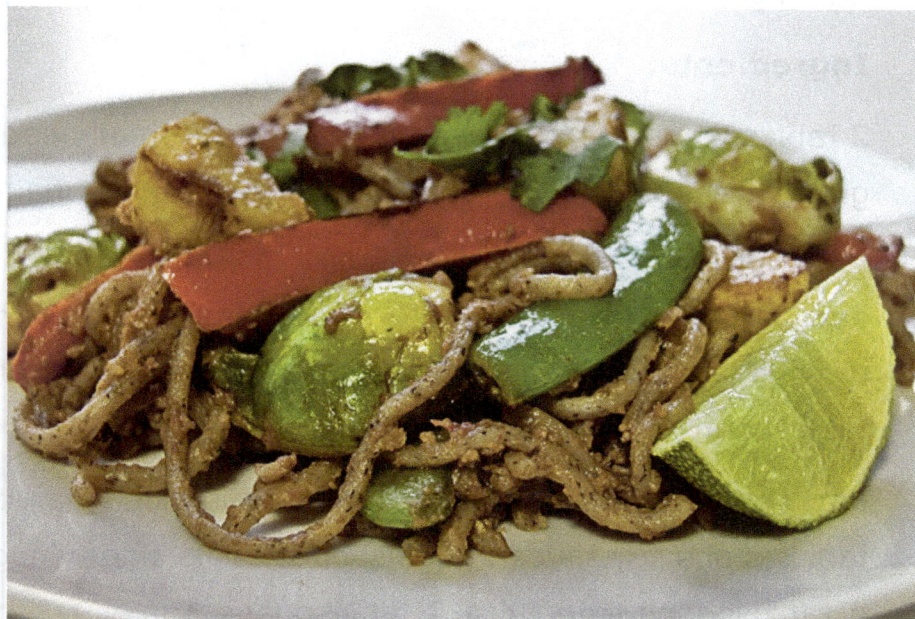

Mango Cabbage Wraps

Preparation time: 15 minutes Cooking time: 35 minutes
Servings: 4

Ingredients:

2 tablespoons chopped peanuts, toasted 1 small head of
green cabbage 2 tablespoons coconut flakes,
unsweetened, toasted

For the Baked Tofu: 15 ounces tofu, extra-firm,
drained, cut into ½-inch cubed 2 teaspoons cornstarch 1
tablespoon soy sauce 1 tablespoon olive oil

For the Peanut Sauce: 1 teaspoon minced garlic 2
tablespoons soy sauce 2 tablespoons apple cider vinegar
4 tablespoons lime juice 2 tablespoons honey 1/3 cup
peanut butter 2 teaspoons toasted sesame oil

For the Mango Pico: 4 green onions, chopped 2
mangos, peeled, stoned, diced 1 medium red bell pepper,
cored, chopped 1 jalapeño, minced 1/3 cup cilantro
leaves, chopped ¼ teaspoon salt 2 tablespoons lime juice

Directions:

Prepare tofu and for this, place tofu pieces on a baking
sheet, drizzle with 1 tablespoon oil and soy sauce, and

toss until coated. Sprinkle with 1 teaspoon cornstarch, toss until incorporated, sprinkle with remaining corn starch, toss until well coated, arrange tofu pieces in a single layer and bake for 35 minutes at 400 degrees F until crispy and golden brown. Meanwhile, prepare the peanut sauce and for this, place all its ingredients in a food processor and pulse for 2 minutes until blended, set aside until required. Prepare the salsa and for this, place all its ingredients in a bowl and toss until mixed. When tofu has baked, take a pan, place it over medium heat, add toast peanuts and coconut flakes in it, and then add tofu pieces. Pour in two-third of the peanut sauce, toss until well coated, cook for 5 minutes until its edges begin to bowl, then transfer tofu to a plate and let cool for 10 minutes. Prepare the wrap and for this, pull out one leaf at a time from the cabbage, add some salsa, top with tofu, drizzle with remaining peanut sauce and serve

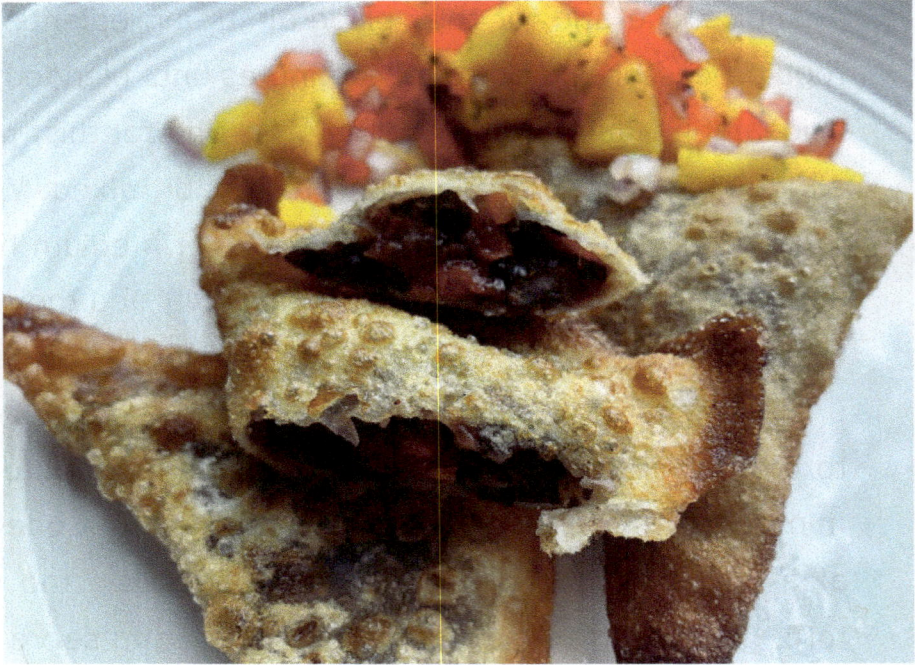

Grilled Asparagus and Shiitake Tacos

Preparation time: 5 minutes Cooking time: 15 minutes
Servings: 4

Ingredients:

8 ounces shiitake mushrooms, destemmed 1 bunch of green onions 2 teaspoons minced garlic 1 teaspoon ground chipotle chili 1/2 teaspoon salt 3 tablespoons olive oil 8 corn tortillas, warmed 4 lime wedges 1 cup guacamole ¼ cup cilantro sprigs 4 tablespoons hot sauce

Directions:

Take a large baking dish, add garlic, salt, and chipotle and stir in oil until combined. Add all the vegetables, toss until well coated, and then grill over medium heat until lightly charred, 6 minutes grilling time for asparagus, 5 minutes for onions and mushrooms. When done, cut vegetables for 2-inch pieces, distribute them evenly between tortillas, top with cilantro, guacamole, and hot sauce and serve with lime wedges.

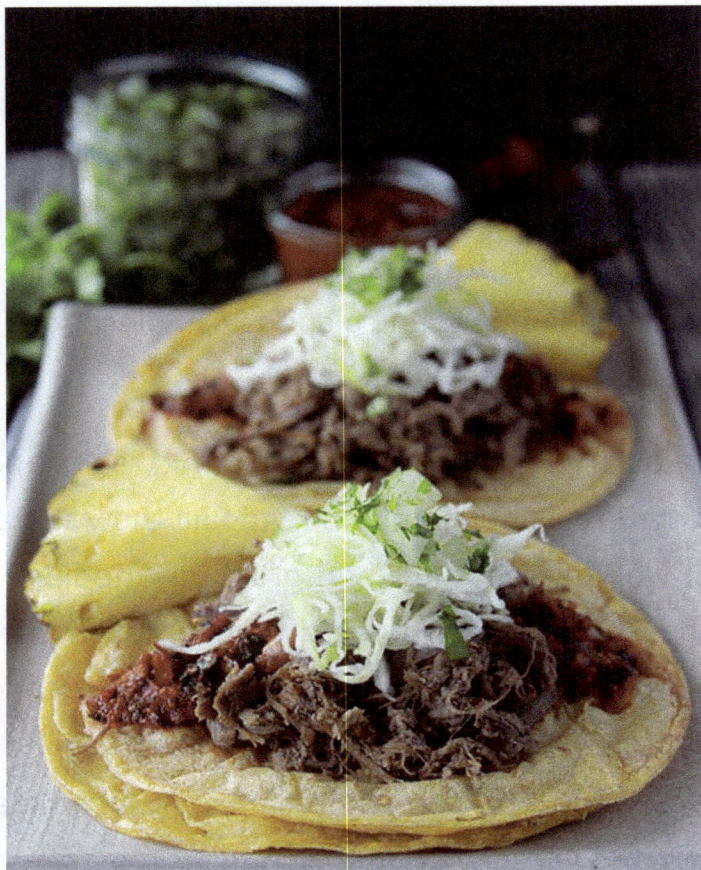

BBQ Chickpea and Cauliflower Flatbreads

Preparation time: 5 minutes Cooking time: 15 minutes Servings: 4

Ingredients:

2 avocados, peeled, pitted, sliced 1 cup BBQ chickpeas 12 ounces chopped cauliflower florets 1 teaspoon salt 2 tablespoons roasted pumpkin seeds, salted 1 tablespoon olive oil 2 tablespoons lemon juice 4 flatbreads, toasted Hot sauce as needed for serving

Directions:

Place a large baking sheer]t, place cauliflower in it, add oil, season with ¼ teaspoon salt, toss until well coated, and then bake for 25 minutes at 425 degrees F until don't. Meanwhile, place the avocado in a bowl, add remaining salt and lemon juice, mash well with a fork and then spread on one side of flatbreads. Distribute roasted cauliflower between flatbreads, top with chickpeas and pumpkin seeds, drizzle with hot sauce and then serve.

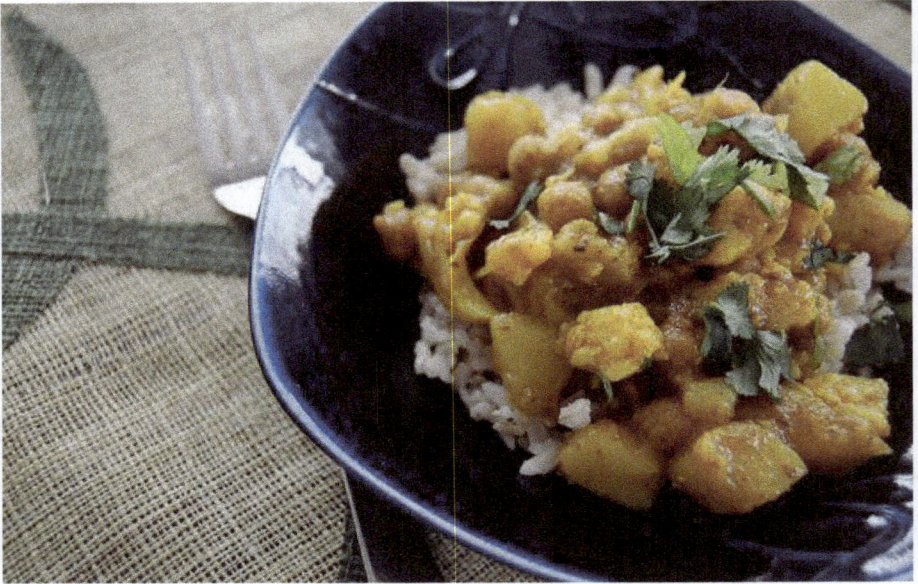

Potatoes with Nacho Sauce

Preparation time: 10 minutes Cooking time: 30 minutes
Servings: 4

Ingredients:

2 pounds mixed baby potatoes, halved 1/2 jalapeno chili, deseeded, chopped 1 cup cashews, soaked, drained 1/2 teaspoon garlic powder 1/2 teaspoon red chili powder 1 teaspoon of sea salt 1/2 teaspoon sweet paprika 1/2 teaspoon ground cumin 1/4 cup nutritional yeast 3 tablespoons lemon juice 3 tablespoons olive oil 1 cup of water Tortilla chips for serving

Directions:

Place potatoes in a baking sheet, drizzle with oil, season with ½ teaspoon salt and ¼ teaspoon black pepper, and roast for 30 minutes at 450 degrees F until crispy and golden. Meanwhile, place the remaining ingredients in a blender and pulse for 2 minutes until smooth. Tip the sauce in a saucepan and cook for 5 minutes at the medium-low level until warm and then serve with roasted potatoes and tortilla chips.

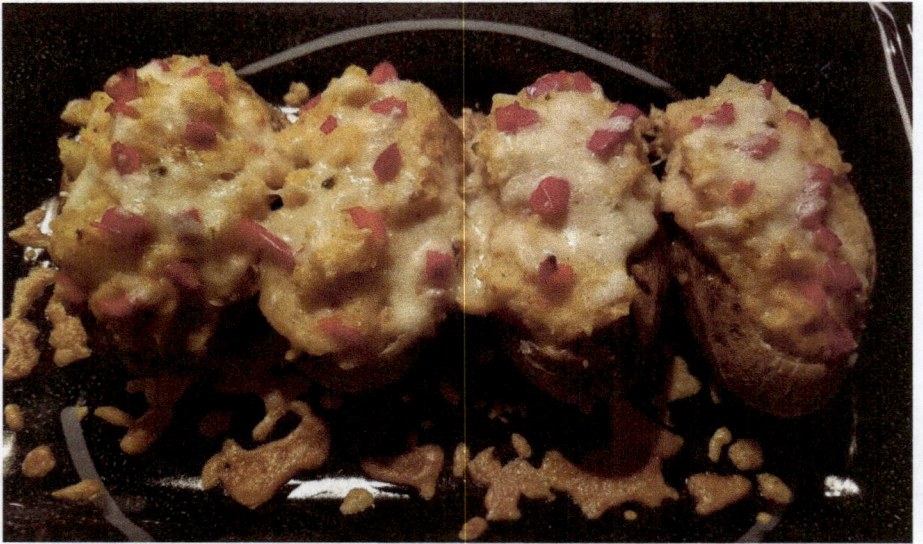

Summer Pesto Pasta

Preparation time: 10 minutes Cooking time: 10 minutes

Servings: 4

Ingredients:

1 pound whole-grain spaghetti, cooked

2 cups grape tomatoes, halved

2 ears corn, shucked

1 medium yellow squash, ½ inch sliced

1 small bell pepper, deseeded, cut into sixths

1 medium zucchini, ½ inch sliced

1/4 cup chopped parsley

 4 green onions

1 teaspoon salt

1 teaspoon ground black pepper

1 lemon, juiced, zested

2 tablespoons olive oil

1/2 cup vegan pesto

Directions: Place corn, onions, bell pepper, zucchini and squash in a bowl, season with ½ teaspoon each of salt and black pepper, and toss until coated. Grill the corn for 10 minutes, and grill remaining vegetables for 6 minutes until lightly charred and when done, chop vegetables and place them in a bowl. Place pesto in another bowl, add lemon juice and zest, season with remaining salt and black pepper, and whisk until combined. Pour pesto over vegetables, toss until mixed, then cut kernels from grilled cobs, add them to the vegetables, then add pasta, parsley, and tomatoes and toss until combined. Serve straight away.

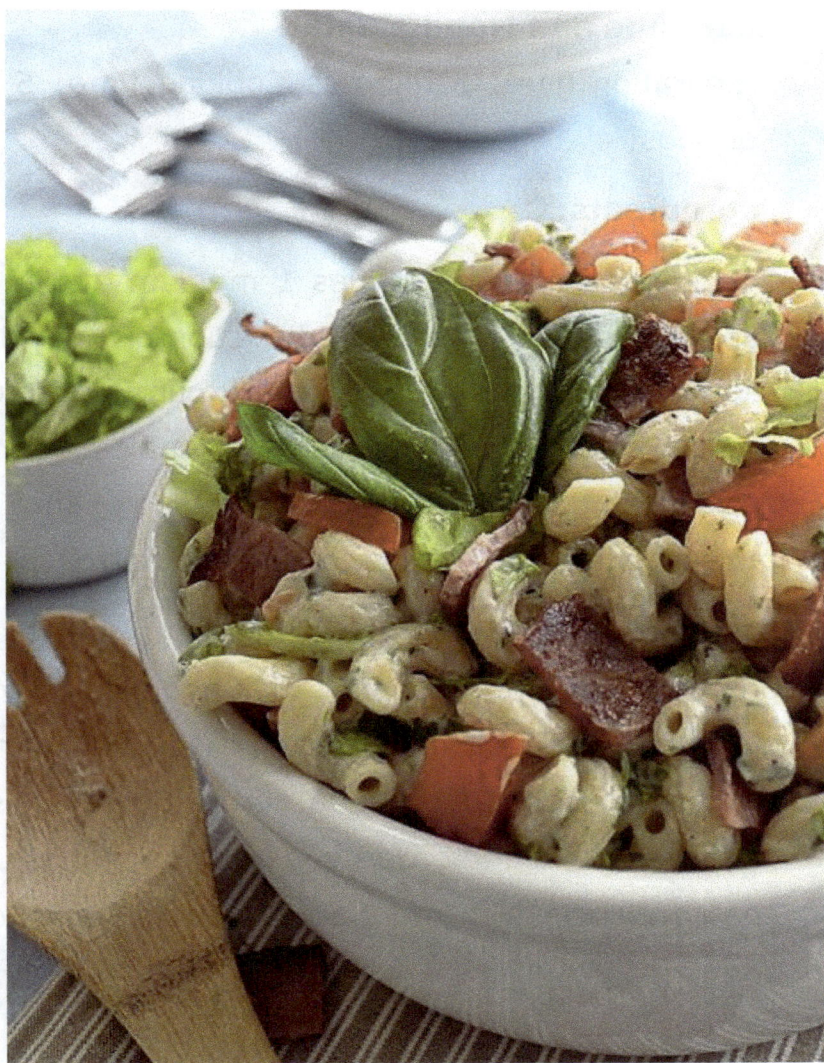

Edamame and Noodle Salad

Preparation time: 5 minutes Cooking time: 5 minutes Servings: 4

Ingredients:

24 ounces shirataki noodles 1 medium apple, sliced 2 cups grape tomatoes, halved 3 cups frozen edamame, shelled 3 cups shredded carrots 2 cups frozen corn 1/2 teaspoon salt 1/2 cup rice vinegar 1 tablespoon Sriracha hot sauce and more for serving 1/2 cup peanut butter 2 tablespoons water 1/2 cup chopped cilantro

Directions: Take a large pot, place it over high heat, pour in water, bring it to boil, then add noodles, corn and edamame, boil for 2 minutes and drain when done. Place remaining ingredients in a large bowl, whisk until combined, then add boiled vegetables and toss until well coated. Drizzle with more Sriracha sauce and toss until combined.

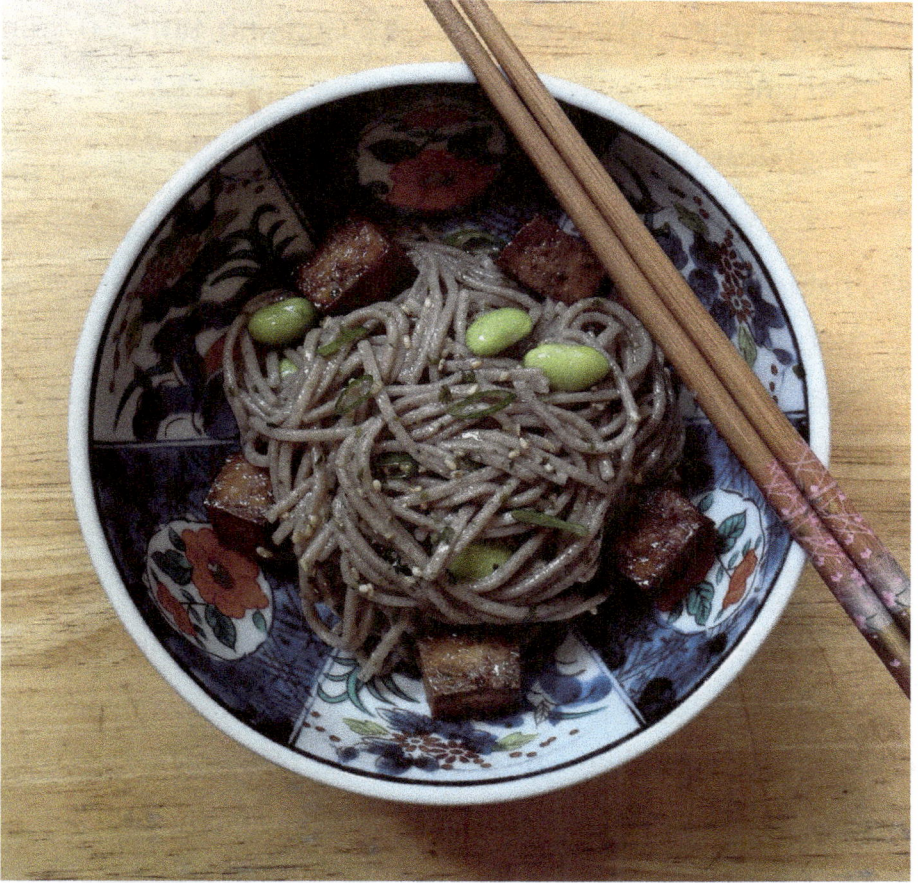

Avocado and Lime Bean Bowl

Preparation time: 10 minutes Cooking time: 0 minute Servings: 1

Ingredients:

1/2 cup mint berries 1/4 of medium avocado, pitted, sliced 1/2 cup breakfast beans 12 ounces roasted vegetable mix 1/8 teaspoon salt 1/8 teaspoon cumin 1 teaspoon sunflower seeds 1 teaspoon lime juice Lime wedges for serving

Directions:

Place avocado in a bowl, mash with a fork and then stir in lime juice, salt, and cumin until combined. Place roasted vegetable mix in a dish, top with mashed avocado mixture, beans, and sunflower seeds. Serve with lime wedges and berries.

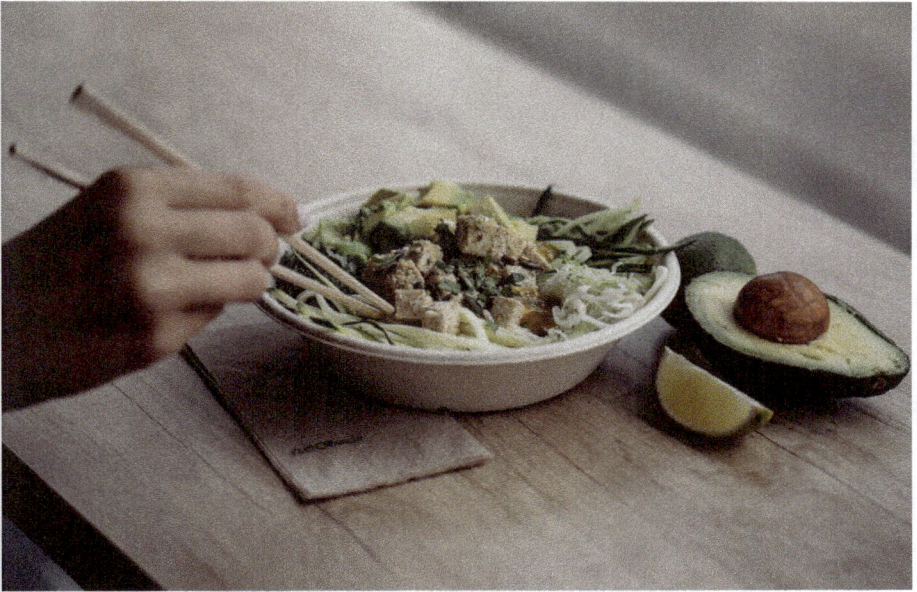

Balsamic-Glazed Roasted Cauliflower

Preparation time:10 minutes Cooking time:1 hour and 5 minutes Servings: 4

Ingredients:

1 large head cauliflower, cut into florets 1/2 pound green beans, trimmed 1 medium red onion, peeled, cut into wedges 2 cups cherry tomatoes ½ teaspoon salt 1/4 cup brown sugar 3 tablespoons olive oil 1 cup balsamic vinegar 2 tablespoons chopped parsley, for garnish

Directions:

Place cauliflower florets in a baking dish, add tomatoes, green beans and onion wedges around it, season with salt, and drizzle with oil. Pour vinegar in a saucepan, stir in sugar, bring the mixture to a boil and simmer for 15 minutes until reduced by half. Brush the sauce generously over cauliflower florets and then roast for 1 hour at 400 degrees F until cooked, brushing sauce frequently. When done, garnish vegetables with parsley and then serve.

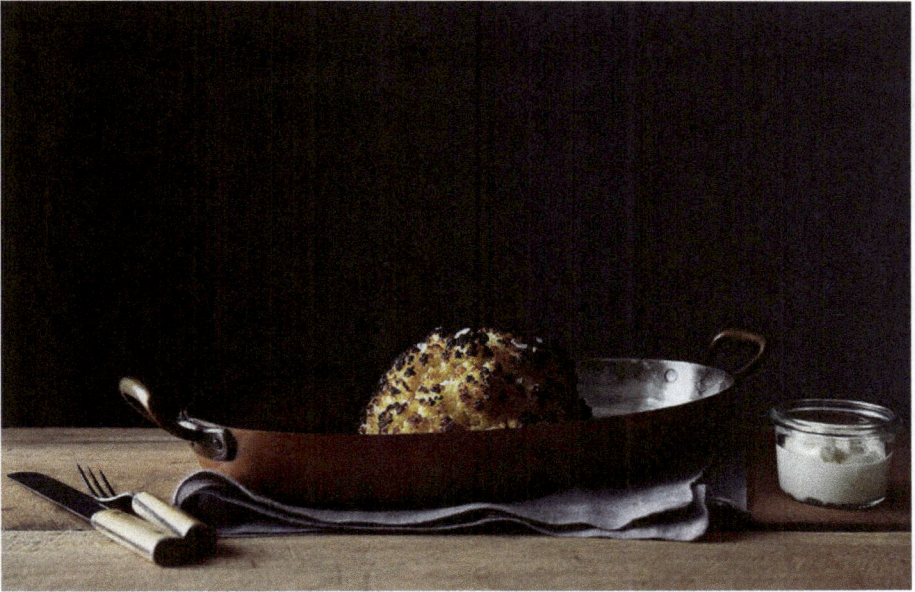

Split Pea Pesto Stuffed Shells

Preparation time: 15 minutes Cooking time: 60 minutes
Servings: 6

Ingredients:

12 ounces jumbo pasta shells, whole-grain, cooked
Marinara sauce as needed for serving

For the Split Pea Pesto:

1 cup green split peas

1/4 cup basil leaves

1 teaspoon minced garlic

1 teaspoon of sea salt

2 tablespoons lemon juice

2 1/4 cups water, divided

Directions:

Take a small saucepan, place it over high heat, add peas, pour in 2 cups water, and bring the beans to boil. Switch heat to the low level, simmer beans for 30 minutes, and when done, drain the beans then transfer them to a food processor. Pour in remaining ingredients for the pesto and pulse until blended. Take a baking dish, spread the marinara sauce in the bottom, then stuffed shell with prepared pesto, arrange them into the prepared baking dish, spread with some marinara sauce over the top and bake for 30 minutes until heated. Garnish with basil and serve.

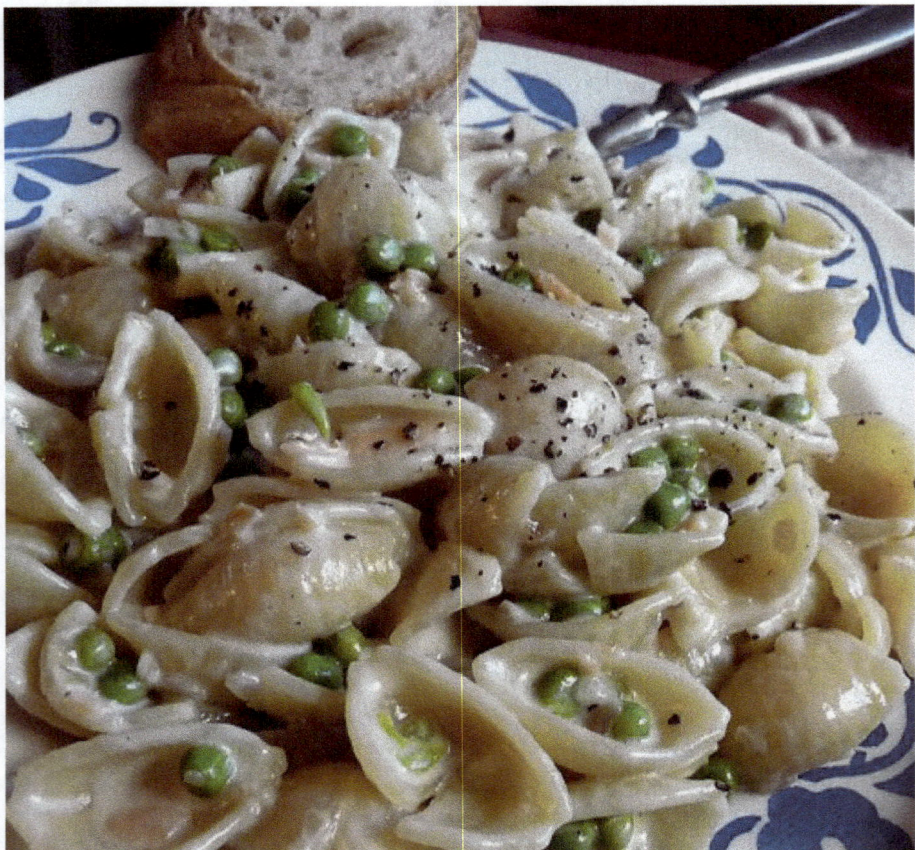

Thai Peanut and Sweet Potato Buddha Bowl

Preparation time: 10 minutes Cooking time: 20 minutes
Servings: 2

Ingredients:

1 cup quinoa, cooked

4 cups sweet potato, peeled, small dice

½ cup carrots shredded

¼ cup cilantro

2 teaspoons minced garlic

2 teaspoons chopped the rosemary

1 teaspoon salt

1 teaspoon ground cinnamon

1 teaspoon ground black pepper

 ¼ cup peanuts, chopped

¼ cup olive oil

½ cup Thai Peanut Sauce

For the Thai Peanut Sauce ¼ cup Thai red curry paste ¼
cup brown sugar 2 tablespoons soy sauce 1 tablespoon

lime juice 1 ½ cups coconut milk 2 tablespoons apple cider vinegar 1 cup peanut butter

Directions:

Place sweet potatoes in a baking dish, add garlic, drizzle with oil, sprinkle with salt, rosemary, black pepper, and cinnamon and bake for 20 minutes at 425 degrees F until roasted. Meanwhile, prepare the peanut sauce, and for this, place all its ingredients in a food processor and pulse until smooth. When sweet potatoes have cooked, distribute them between two bowls along with peanuts, quinoa, cilantro, and carrots and then drizzle with sauce generously. Serve straight away

Meatball Sub

Preparation time: 10 minutes Cooking time: 22 minutes
Servings: 3

Ingredients:

For the Meatballs: 1/3 cup sunflower seeds, ground

1 1/2 cups cooked kidney beans

1/2 cup mushrooms, chopped

1/2 cup rolled oats ½ teaspoon minced garlic

1 small red onion, peeled, chopped

2/3 teaspoon salt

1 teaspoon dried oregano

1/3 teaspoon ground black pepper

1 teaspoon dried basil

1 teaspoon soy sauce

1 tablespoon olive oil

1 tablespoon tomato paste

For the Subs: 3 Italian sub rolls 1/4 cup chopped parsley
2 cups marinara sauce 3 tablespoons grated vegan Parmesan

Directions:

Place beans in a bowl, mash them with a fork and set aside until required. Then place a medium pan over medium heat, add oil and when hot, add onions, cook for 3 minutes, stir in garlic and mushrooms and cook for another 2 minutes. Then stir in mashed beans, add oats, sunflower seeds, tomato paste, all the spices and soy sauce, stir until well combined, and shape the mixture into 14 meatballs. Arrange meatballs onto a baking sheet lined with parchment paper and bake for 15 minutes at 350 degrees F until cooked. Sandwich the meatballs evenly between sub rolls, top with marinara, parmesan cheese, and parsley, and then serve.

White Bean and Mushroom Meatballs Subs

Preparation time: 15 minutes Cooking time: 30 minutes Servings: 20

Ingredients:

For The Meatballs:

1 1/4 cups bread crumbs

15 ounces cooked white beans

1 small white onion, peeled, diced

8 ounces button mushrooms, chopped

1 teaspoon minced garlic

1/2 teaspoon ground black pepper

1 teaspoon salt

1/2 teaspoon red chili flake

1 teaspoon oregano

1 lemon, juiced

1 tablespoon olive oil

2 tablespoons parsley, chopped

For the Subs: 15 ounces marinara sauce 20 sub rolls

Directions: Take a large skillet pan, place it over medium heat, add oil and when hot, add onion and cook for 5 minutes. Then add garlic and mushrooms, cook for 2 minutes, add beans, season with salt, red chili flakes, oregano, and black pepper, stir in lemon juice and cook for 1 minute. Transfer the mixture into the food processor, puree until smooth, add 1 cup crumbs and parsley and pulse until well combined. Let the mixture stand for five minutes, shape the mixture into twenty meatballs, cover with remaining breadcrumbs until coated, and cook for 20 minutes until nicely browned on all sides. Sandwich the meatballs in sub rolls, top with marinara sauce and serve.

Vegetarian Biryani

Preparation time: 10 minutes Cooking time: 33 minutes
Servings: 6

Ingredients:

12 ounces chickpeas

2 cups rice, rinsed

1 large onion, peeled, sliced

2 cups sliced mixed veggies

1 ½ teaspoon minced garlic

1 tablespoon grated ginger

1 tablespoon cumin

1/2 teaspoon turmeric

1 tablespoon coriander

3/4 teaspoon salt

1 teaspoon cinnamon

1 teaspoon red chili powder

1/2 teaspoon cardamom

1 bay leaf 1/2 cup raisins

2 tablespoons olive oil

4 cups vegetable stock Garnishing

1/4 cup cashews

1/4 cup chopped parsley

Directions: Take a large skillet pan, place it over medium-high heat, add oil and when hot, add onion and cook for 5 minutes. Then add vegetables, ginger, and garlic, continue cooking for 5 minutes, reserve 1 cup of the mixture and set it aside. Add bay leaf into the pan, stir in all the spices, cook for 1 minute, stir in rice and cook for 1 minute. Season with salt, pour in the stock, then top with reserved vegetables, chickpeas and raisins, switch heat to a high level, and bring the mixture to simmer. Then switch heat to the low level, cover the pan with a towel, place lid on top of it to seal the pan completely, and simmer for 20 minutes until all the liquid has soaked by the rice. When done, fluff the rice with a fork, top with cilantro and cashews, and then serve.

Chinese Eggplant with Szechuan Sauce

Preparation time: 10 minutes Cooking time: 25 minutes Servings: 4

Ingredients:

1 1/2 pound Eggplant

2 teaspoons minced garlic

2 teaspoons grated ginger

2 tablespoons cornstarch

2 teaspoons salt

4 tablespoons peanut oil

10 dried red chilies

For the Szechuan Sauce: 1 teaspoon Szechuan peppercorns, toasted, crushed 1/2 teaspoon five-spice 1 tablespoon mirin 3 tablespoons brown sugar 1 teaspoon red chili flakes 1/4 cup soy sauce 1 tablespoon rice vinegar 1 tablespoon sesame oil

Directions: Cut eggplant into bite-size pieces, place them in a large bowl, cover them with water, stir in salt and let them stand for 15 minutes. Prepare the Szechuan sauce and for this, place all its ingredients in a small bowl except for Szechuan peppercorns and whisk until combined and set aside until required. Pat dry eggplant with paper towels, sprinkle with corn starch and then fry them in a single layer over medium heat for 10 minutes until golden brown. When eggplants are done, transfer them to a plate, add some more oil into the pan, add garlic and ginger and cook for 2 minutes. Add Szechuan peppercorns and prepared sauce, stir until combined and simmer for 20 seconds. Return eggplant pieces into the pan, toss until mixed, cook for 1 minute and then garnish with green onions. Serve straight away.

Ramen with Miso Shiitake

Preparation time: 10 minutes Cooking time: 35 minutes
Servings: 4

Ingredients:

For Ramen Broth: 1 large white onion, peeled, diced

1/3 teaspoon ground black pepper

1/2 cup dried Shiitake Mushrooms, chopped

2 tablespoons white miso paste

1 teaspoon minced garlic

2 tablespoons olive oil

1/8 cup mirin

4 cups vegetable stock

4 cups of water

For the Ramen: 8 ounces cubed tofu, crispy as needed
8 ounces cooked ramen noodles as needed Sautéed bok
choy as needed Fresh spinach as needed Shredded

carrots as needed Roasted winter squash as needed Roasted cauliflower as needed Roasted carrots as needed Roasted sweet potato as needed Sautéed mushrooms as needed Smoked mushrooms as needed Pickled radish as needed Mix herbs as needed

For Garnish: Scallions as needed Sesame seeds as needed Sriracha as needed Sesame oil as needed

Directions: Prepare the broth and for this, place a pot over medium-high heat, add 1 tablespoon oil and when hot, add onion and cook for 3 minutes. Switch heat to medium level, stir in garlic, cook for 1 minute, then add remaining ingredients for the broth and simmer for 30 minutes until done. Distribute all the ingredients for ramen evenly between four bowls, then pour in broth and top evenly with garnishing ingredients. Serve straight away.

Tofu with Bok Choy

Preparation time: 10 minutes Cooking time: 15 minutes Servings: 2

Ingredients:

6 ounces baby bok choy, quartered lengthwise

12 ounces tofu, firm, drained, cut it into 1-inch cubes 1 shallot, peeled, sliced

2 teaspoons minced garlic

1 teaspoon ground black pepper ¼ teaspoon salt

2 tablespoons peanut oil Corn starch as needed for dredging

For the Black Pepper Sauce: ½ teaspoon ground black pepper 2 tablespoons soy sauce 1 teaspoon brown sugar 2 tablespoons of rice wine 1 teaspoon red chili paste 2 tablespoons water

Directions: Prepare the sauce and for this, take a skillet pan, add all the ingredients in it and whisk until combined. Take another skillet pan, place it over medium-high heat, add 1 tablespoon peanut oil and when hot, add salt and black pepper and cook for 1 minute. Dredge tofu pieces in cornstarch, add them into the skillet pan, and cook for 6 minutes until seared and crispy on all sides. When done, transfer tofu pieces to a plate lined with paper towels and set aside until required. Add remaining oil into the pan and when hot, add bok choy, shallots and garlic, stir and cook for 4 minutes. Pour in the prepared sauce, toss until mixed and simmer for 3 minutes until bok choy is tender. Then add crispy tofu pieces, toss until coated, cook for 3 minutes until heated, and then serve.

Veggie Lo Mein

Preparation time: 5 minutes Cooking time: 15 minutes Servings: 2

Ingredients:

5 ounces lo mein noodles or whole-wheat linguine, cooked

For the Lo Mein Sauce:

1/8 teaspoon ground white pepper 1 teaspoon sriracha 1 teaspoon maple syrup 1/4 teaspoon liquid smoke 1 tablespoon oyster sauce 3 tablespoons soy sauce 2 tablespoons Chinese cooking wine 2 teaspoons sesame oil

For the Lo Mein Stir Fry:

1/2 a white onion, peeled, sliced 1 teaspoon grated ginger 2 cups sliced mushrooms 1 ½ teaspoon minced garlic 1 cup shredded cabbage 1/2 of medium red bell pepper, sliced 1 cup carrot, cut into matchstick 1 cup snow peas ¼ cup baby spinach ¼ cup bok choy ¼ cup shredded Brussel sprouts ¼ cup bean sprouts 2 tablespoons peanut oil

For the Garnish:

Scallions, sliced, as needed

Directions:

Prepare the sauce and for this, place all its ingredients in a small bowl and whisk until combined. Take a large skillet pan, place it over medium-high heat, add oil and when hot, add onion and mushrooms and cook for 4 minutes, stirring constantly. Switch heat to medium level, add garlic and ginger, cook for 2 minutes, then add remaining vegetables and continue cooking for 4 minutes until crispy. Add noodles, toss until mixed, stir in the sauce until coated, cook for 2 minutes until hot and then divide evenly between bowls. Top with scallions and serve.

Middle Eastern Salad Tacos

Preparation time: 10 minutes Cooking time: 5 minutes
Servings: 3

Ingredients:

For the Spiced Chickpeas:

12 ounces cooked chickpeas

½ cup hummus

½ teaspoon salt

1 teaspoon cumin

1 teaspoon sumac

2 teaspoons olive oil

1 teaspoon sesame seeds

6 tortillas, warmed, about

6-inches Scallions for topping

For the Salad:

2 cucumbers, diced

1 tomato, diced

½ cup arugula

¼ teaspoon salt

1 teaspoon ground coriander

2 tablespoons olive oil

2 tablespoons lemon juice

Directions:

Take a skillet pan, place it over medium heat, add oil and when hot, add chickpeas, stir in salt and all the spices and cook for 3 minutes until warm. When done, remove the pan from heat, sprinkle with sesame seeds and set aside. Take a bowl, place all the ingredients for the salad in it, and toss until mixed. Spread hummus on one side of the tortilla, top with chickpeas and salad, sprinkle with scallion, and then serve

Zaatar Roasted Eggplant

Preparation time: 10 minutes Cooking time: 60 minutes Servings: 2

Ingredients:

1 pound eggplant, destemmed ½ teaspoon minced garlic ¼ teaspoon salt 1 tablespoon zaatar spice mix 1 ½ tablespoon olive oil For Serving: 2 cups chopped tomatoes 2 cups cooked brown rice Tahini sauce as needed Parsley for serving

Directions: Prepare the eggplant, and for this, cut it into half, then make deep diagonals in it at 1-inch interval, but not cutting through the skin and season with 1/8 teaspoon salt. Place remaining ingredients in a bowl, stir until the smooth paste comes together, then brush it well on the eggplant, bake for 1 hour until tender, rotating halfway, and when done, pierce it with a fork. When done, top eggplant with rice and tomatoes, drizzle with tahini sauce, top with parsley and serve.

Vegetarian fajitas

Preparation time: 10 minutes Cooking time: 15 minutes
Servings: 6

Ingredients:

For the Vegetables:

12 ounces cooked black beans

1 yellow bell pepper, cored, sliced

2 green bell peppers, cored, sliced

1 medium-sized white onion, peeled, sliced

1 red bell pepper, cored, sliced 3

 tablespoons olive oil

For the Fajita Seasoning:

1/2 teaspoon onion powder

1/2 teaspoon garlic powder

1/2 teaspoon ground black pepper

1/2 teaspoon salt

2 teaspoons red chili powder

1/8 teaspoon cayenne pepper 1 teaspoon paprika

For the Toppings: 6 small tortillas Guacamole as needed

1 lime, cut into wedges

2 tablespoons chopped cilantro

Directions: Prepare the fajita seasoning and for this, stir all its ingredients, then sprinkle with over onion and bell peppers, drizzle with oil, toss until well coated, spread them evenly on a sheet pan and bake for 15 minutes until roasted, tossing halfway. When done, heat beans over low heat until hot, then distribute it evenly on the tortilla, top with roasted vegetables, guacamole, and cilantro and serve with lime wedges.

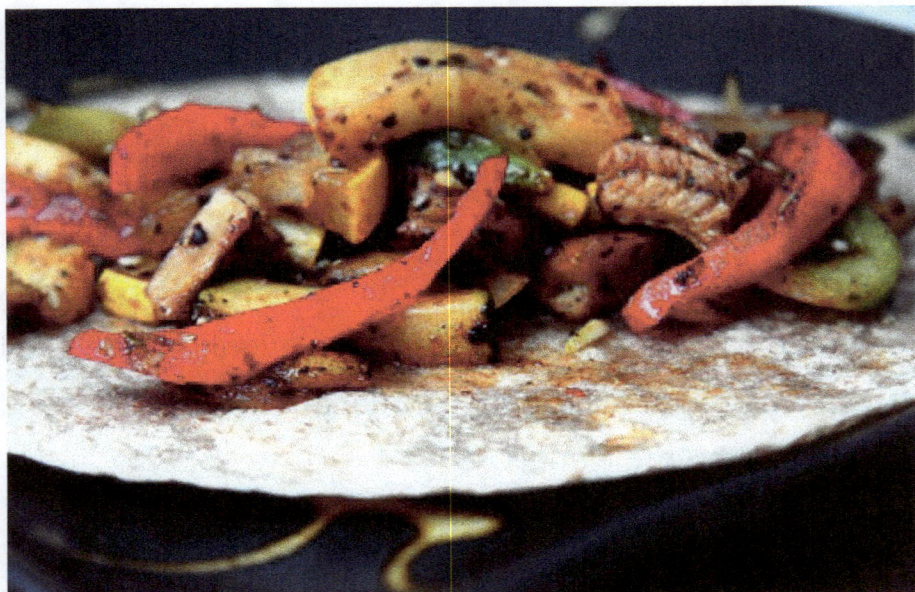

Tikka Masala with Cauliflower

Preparation time: 10 minutes Cooking time: 22 minutes Servings: 4

Ingredients:

1 medium head of cauliflower, cut into small florets 1 medium shallot, peeled, chopped 1 medium red bell pepper, cored, diced 2 teaspoons minced garlic 2 medium tomatoes, diced 1 tablespoon grated ginger 1 teaspoon salt ½ teaspoon red chili powder 1 teaspoon curry powder 1 teaspoon turmeric 1 teaspoon cumin 1 teaspoon coriander 1 teaspoon fenugreek leaves 1 lemon, juiced 2 tablespoons olive oil 12 ounces coconut milk, unsweetened 2 tablespoons chopped cilantro

Directions: Take a large pot, place it over medium-high heat, add oil and when hot, add shallot, ginger, and garlic and cook for 3 minutes. Switch heat to medium level, add all the spices and seeds, cook for 2 minutes, then stir in tomatoes and cook for 2 minutes. Pour in milk, stir until incorporated, bring the mixture to simmer, switch heat to medium-low level, add bell pepper and florets, stir until mixed and simmer for 12 minutes until tender. Stir in lemon juice and serve straight away.

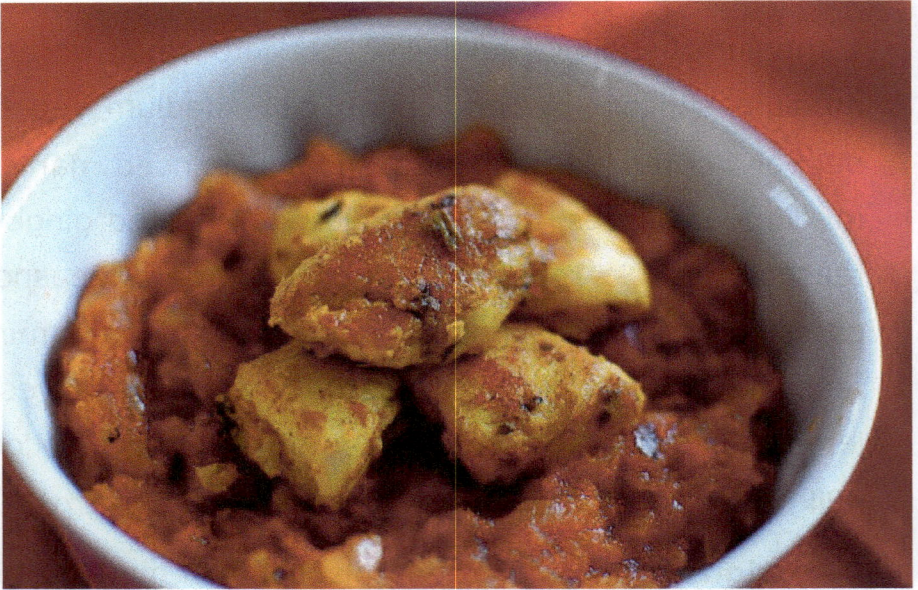

Sweetcorn and Zucchini Fritters

Preparation time: 10 minutes Cooking time: 20 minutes
Servings: 2

Ingredients: 1 1/2 cups corn kernels, cooked 4 cups shredded zucchini 3/4 cup chopped green onions 1 1/4 cup chickpea flour 1 ½ teaspoon minced garlic 1 teaspoon salt 1 teaspoon dried oregano 1 teaspoon dried thyme 2 teaspoons cumin ½ teaspoon ground black pepper 2 tablespoons olive oil Salsa for serving

Directions:

Place all the ingredients in a large bowl, except for oil and salsa, stir until well combined, and let it stand for 5 minutes. Take a large skillet pan, place it over medium heat, add oil and when hot, scoop ¼ cup of zucchini mixture per fritter in the pan and cook for 5 minutes per side until golden brown. When done, serve fritters with salsa.

Spiced Carrot and Lentil Soup

Preparation time: 5 minutes Cooking time: 20 minutes
Servings: 4

Ingredients:

22 ounces carrots, grated 5 ounces split red lentils ½ teaspoon salt 2 teaspoons cumin seeds, toasted 1/8 teaspoon red chili flakes 2 tablespoons olive oil 4 cups vegetable stock, hot ½ cup of coconut milk

Directions:

Take a large saucepan, add 1 teaspoon cumin seeds, half of the red chili flakes along with remaining ingredients, stir until combined, and bring the mixture to a boil over medium-high heat. Switch heat to medium level, simmer for 15 minutes until lentils have softened, and when done, puree the soup by using an immersion blender until smooth. Serve straight away.

Tomato and Basil Sauce

Preparation time: 5 minutes Cooking time: 10 minutes
Servings: 4

Ingredients:

14 ounces chopped tomatoes ½ teaspoon minced garlic
1 teaspoon vegetable stock powder 1 teaspoon sugar 1
tablespoon tomato purée 5 basil leaves 1 tablespoon
olive oil ¼ cup vegetable stock

Directions:

Take a skillet pan, place it over medium heat, add oil and
when hot, add garlic and cook for 1 minute until fragrant.
Then stir in tomatoes and remaining ingredients until
combined, except for basil, and bring the mixture to boil.
Switch heat to the low level, simmer the mixture for 5
minutes, and when done, top with basil. Serve straight
away.

Chocolate Fudge

Preparation Time: 10 minutes Serves: 12

Ingredients:

4 oz unsweetened dark chocolate 3/4 cup coconut butter
15 drops liquid stevia 1 tsp vanilla extract

Directions:

Melt coconut butter and dark chocolate. Add Ingredients to the large bowl and combine well. Pour mixture into a silicone loaf pan and place in refrigerator until set. Cut into pieces and serve.

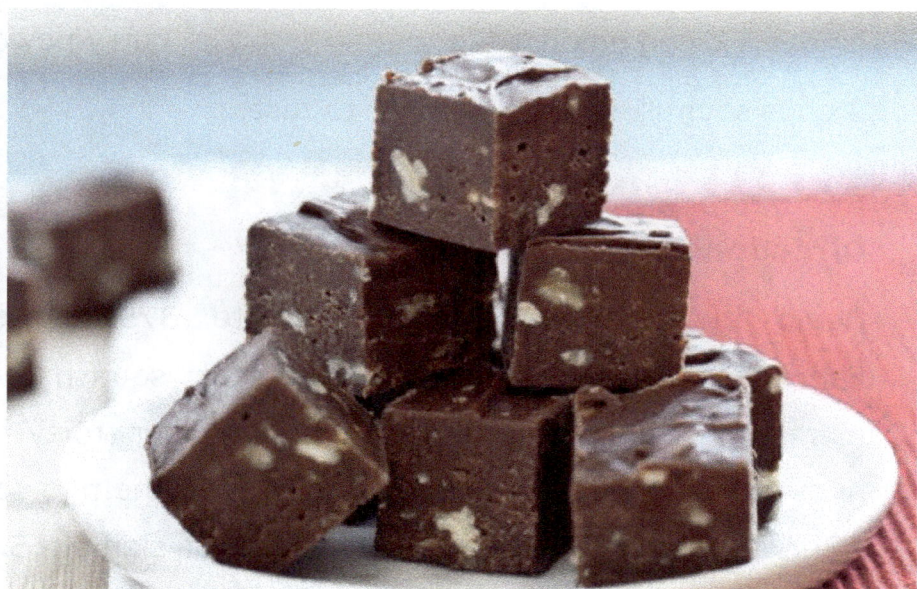

Autumnal Apple and Squash Soup

Preparation time: 5 minutes Cooking time: 60 minutes 6 Servings.

Ingredients:

2 pounds diced butternut squash 2 tbsp. olive oil 3 diced and peeled apples 32 ounces vegetable broth 3 tsp. ginger 1 diced onion 1 tsp. cumin 1 ½ tsp. curry powder 2 cups soymilk salt and pepper to taste

Directions:

Begin by preheating your oven to 375 degrees Fahrenheit. Next, wrap the butternut squash with aluminum foil, and bake the squash for forty-five minutes. Next, set them to the side to allow them to cool. Afterwards, remove the seeds, and peel the skin off. Slice and dice the squash. Bring the squash and the soymilk together in a food processor, and pulse the ingredients. Next, pour the oil into the bottom of the soup pot. Add the onion and sauté the onion for five minutes. Next, add the apple, the broth, and the spices. Bring this mixture to a boil and then allow it to simmer on low for twelve minutes. Next, puree this soup pot mixture in the blender or food processor, and place this back in the soup pot.

Add the squash and the soymilk to the mixture, and stir well. Now, allow this soup to simmer for ten more minutes, and salt and pepper before serving. Enjoy.

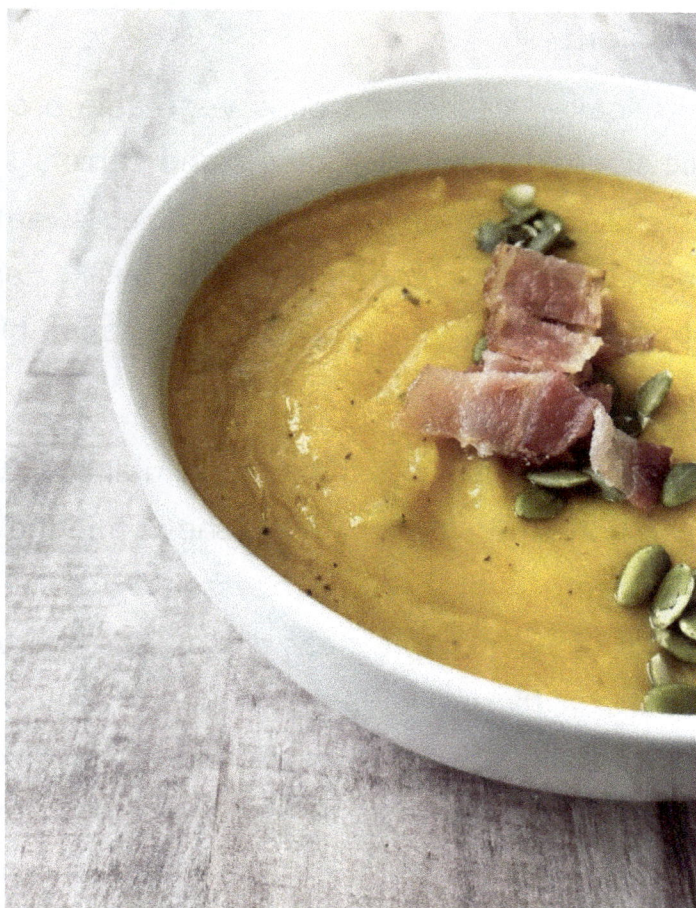

Spicy Vegetable Soup

Preparation time: 5 minutes Cooking time: 20 minutes 6 Servings.

Ingredients:

1 cup soaked cashews 5 cups vegetable broth 3 diced garlic cloves 1 tbsp. olive oil 4 diced carrots 1 diced red pepper 2 chopped celery stalks 1 diced sweet potato 1 28-ounce can diced tomatoes 1 tsp. basil 1 tsp. paprika 1 tsp. cumin 2 cups spinach 15 ounce can of black beans

Directions:

Begin by soaking the cashews in a small bowl with water for two hours. Next, bring the cashews and the vegetable broth together in a food processor. Puree the mixture until it's smooth. Next, heat the oil and the vegetables together for five minutes in a soup pot. Add the spices, and stir, cooking for about seven minutes. Next, add the vegetable broth, and continue to stir. Allow the soup to simmer for twenty minutes. Next, salt and pepper the mixture, and serve the soup warm. Enjoy!

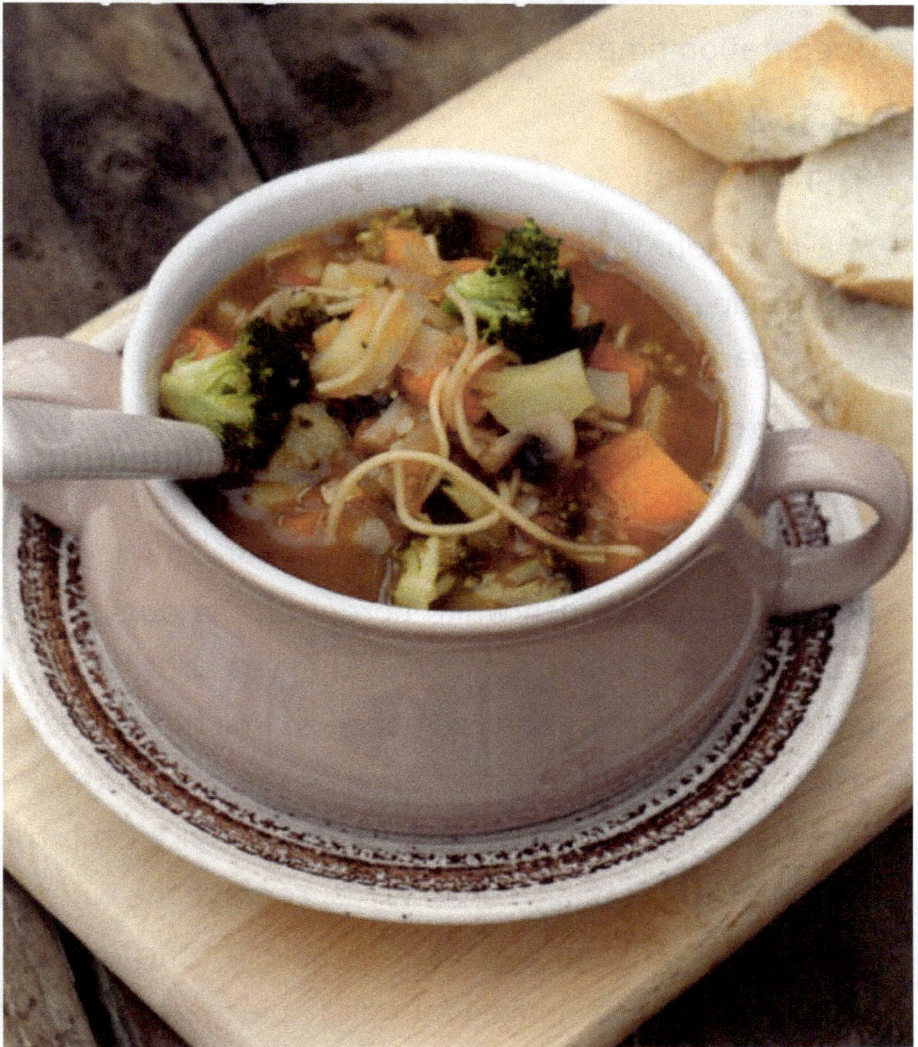

Bean and Carrot Spirals

Preparation time: 10 minutes Cooking time: 40 minutes 24 servings.

Ingredients:

4 8-inch flour tortillas 1 ½ cups of Easy Mean White Bean dip (recipe found here) 10 ounces spinach leaves ½ cup diced carrots ½ cup diced red peppers

Directions:

Begin by preparing the bean dip, seen above. Next, spread out the bean dip on each tortillas, making sure to leave about a ¾ inch white border on the outside of the tortillas. Next, place spinach in the center of the tortilla, followed by carrots and red peppers. Roll the tortillas into tight rolls, and then cover each of the rolls with plastic wrap or aluminum foil. Allow them to chill in the fridge for twenty-four hours. Afterwards, remove the wrap from the spirals and remove the very ends of the rolls. Slice the rolls into six individual spiral pieces, and arrange them on a platter for serving. Enjoy!

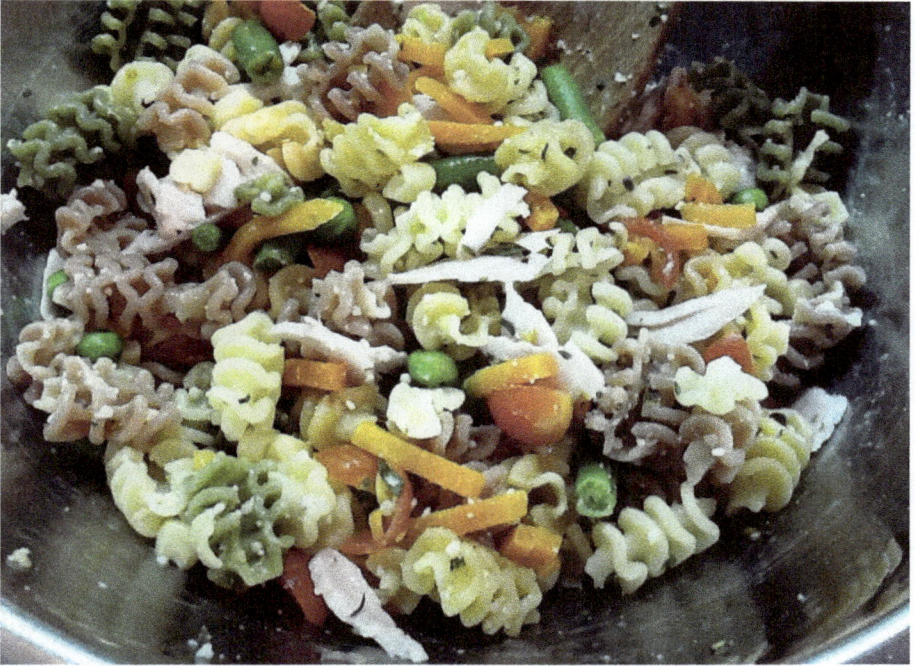

Very Vegan Crunchy Chile Nachos

Preparation time: 10 minutes Cooking time: 50 minutes 8 Servings.

Ingredients:

14 corn tortillas. 1 minced onion 2 tsp. olive oil 1 diced tomato 1 diced garlic 1 tbsp. white flour 2 diced jalapeno peppers 4 tbsp. rice milk 7 ounce grated nondairy cheddar cheese

Directions:

Begin by preheating the oven to 375 degrees Fahrenheit. Next, slice each of the corn tortillas into wedges and place them out on a baking sheet. Allow them to bake for twenty minutes. Afterwards, remove the chips and allow them to cool. Heat garlic and onion together in some olive oil and sauté them for five minutes. Afterwards, add the tomatoes and the jalapenos, and continue to cook and stir for one minute. Add the rice milk. Next, pour the nondairy cheese into the mixture, and stir the ingredients together until the cheese completely melts. Remove the skillet form the heat. Spread out the tortillas on a large plate, and pour the created cheese sauce overtop the chips. Serve warm.

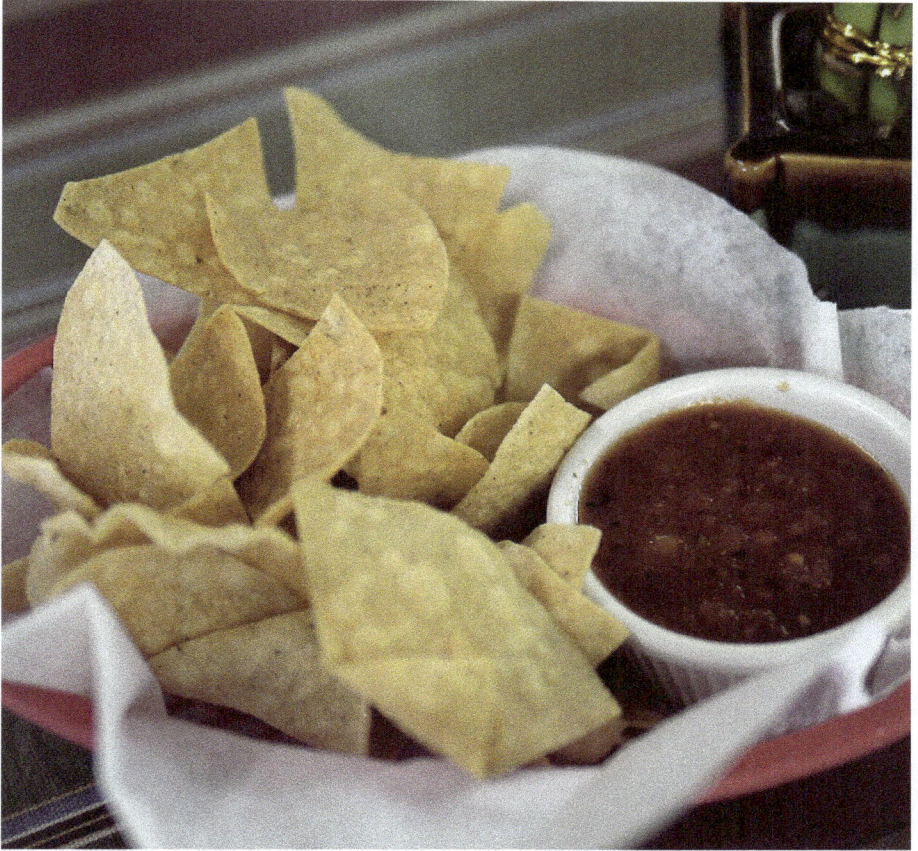

Tofu Nuggets with Barbecue Glaze

9 Servings.

Ingredients:

32 ounces tofu 1 cup quick vegan barbecue sauce

Directions:

Begin by preheating the oven to 425 degrees Fahrenheit. Next, slice the tofu and blot the tofu with clean towels. Next, slice and dice the tofu and completely eliminate the water from the tofu material. Stir the tofu with the vegan barbecue sauce, and place the tofu on a baking sheet. Bake the tofu for fifteen minutes. Afterwards, stir the tofu and bake the tofu for an additional ten minutes. Enjoy!

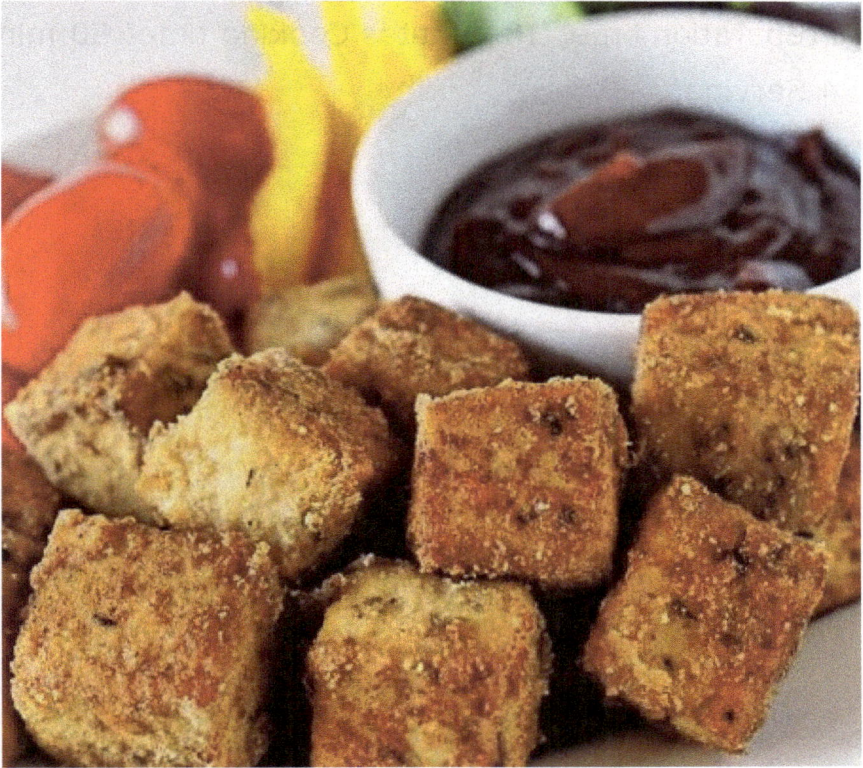

Broiled Japanese Eggplants

Preparation time: 10 minutes Cooking time: 50 minutes
4 Servings.

Ingredients:

2 tbsp. white wine

2 tbps. Sweet rice wine

3 tbsp. agave netar

4 tbsp. mellow white miso

4 Japanese eggplants, sliced in half, de-stemmed

Directions:

Begin by simmering the sweet rice wine and the white wine together in a saucepan. Simmer them together for two minutes. Afterwards, add the miso and stir the ingredients until they're smooth. Add the agave nectar.

At this time, reduce the stovetop heat to low. Continue to heat this mixture while you initiate the next step. Next, place the eggplants with their cut-sides down onto the baking sheet. Place the baking sheet in the broiler for three minutes. Make sure that they do not burn. After three minutes, flip them and cook them for an additional three minutes. The tops should be brown. After the eggplants have cooked, layer the created sauce overtop of them. Place them in the broiler for about forty-five seconds. Afterwards, remove the eggplants and serve them warm. Enjoy!

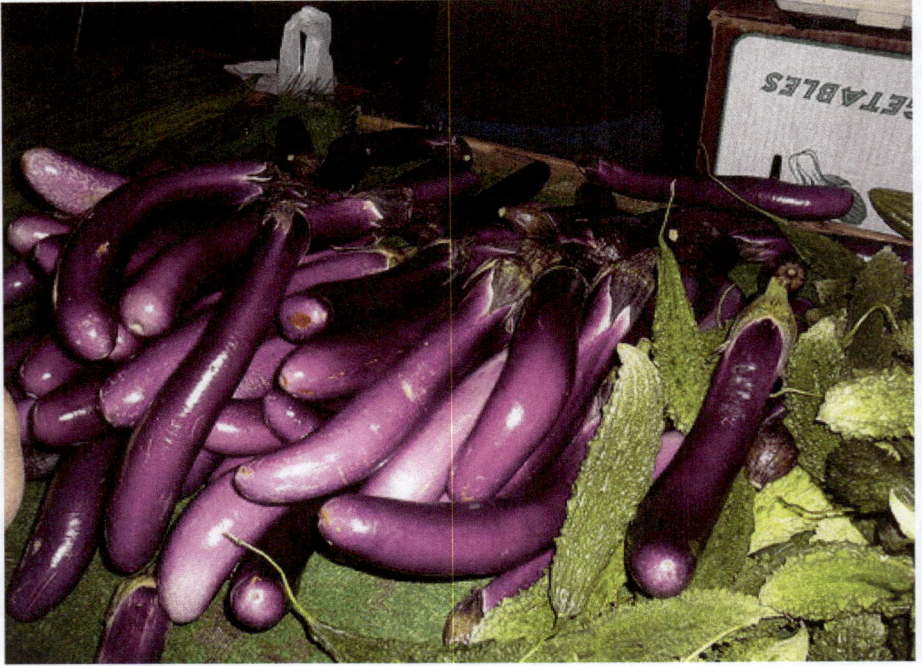

Groovy Indian Samosas

Preparation time: 10 minutes Cooking time: 30 minutes 4 Servings.

Ingredients:

¼ cup olive oil

2 diced onions

1 tsp. mustard seeds

½ tsp. salt

3 tsp. curry powder

1 diced carrot

2 diced potatoes

1 cup diced green beans

1 cup frozen peas

1/3 cup water

8 ounces phyllo pastry sunflower or olive oil for frying

Directions:

Begin by warming up the olive oil in a skillet, and adding the mustard seeds, allowing them to heat until they pop. Add the onions, and cook them for five minutes. Next, pour in the curry powder and the salt. Fry these together for one and a half minutes. Next, add the carrots, the potatoes, the peas, the beans, and the water. Cook this mixture together for fifteen minutes on LOW. The vegetables should be soft. Next, slice up the phyllo pastry to create long strips. Take one strip and place a tbsp.. of the created filling in the strip, at the end. Fold this strip diagonally to create a triangle. Continue this folding until the very end of the strip. Afterwards, seal up the end with water. Repeat the above steps with all the remaining phyllo strips. Afterwards, half-fill a wok with sunflower oil. Heat the oil to 350 degrees Fahrenheit. Next, fry up the samosas for three minutes until they reach a golden color. Allow them to drain, and then serve them warm. Enjoy!

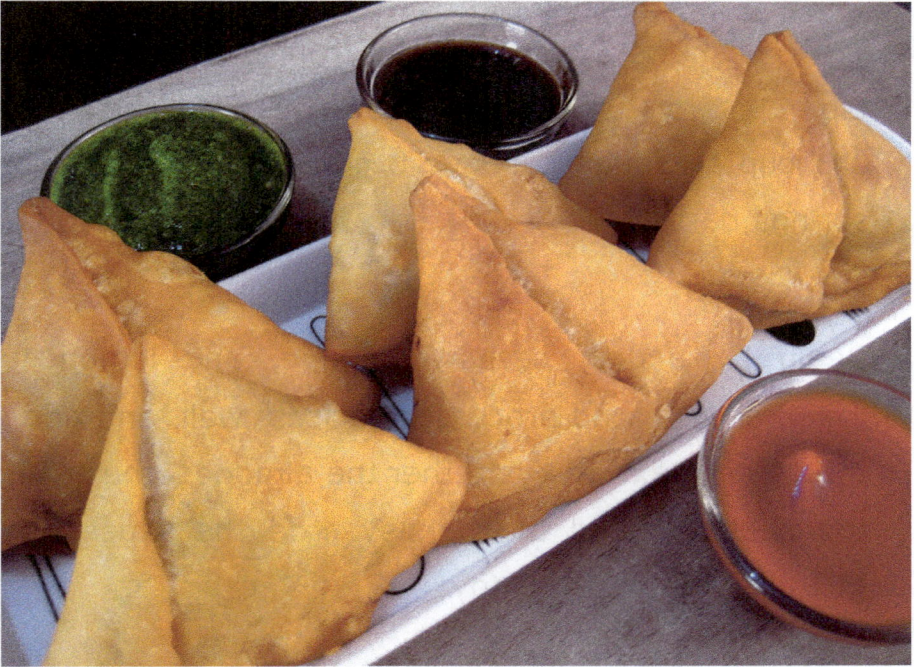

Vegan Creation Coleslaw

Preparation time: 10 minutes Cooking time: 30 minutes 3 cups.

Ingredients:

1 cup cashews 2 tbsp. agave syrup juice of 2 lemons 1 tsp. mustard 1 tsp. Dijon mustard 1/3 cup sliced almonds 1/3 cup shredded cabbage 3 cups shredded spinach 4 springs parsley

Directions:

Begin by adding cashews, agave, and lemon juice together in a food processor. Process well, and add the mustards. Next, mix together the almonds, the spinach, the cabbage, and the parsley. Add the sauce to the mixture, and serve. Enjoy!

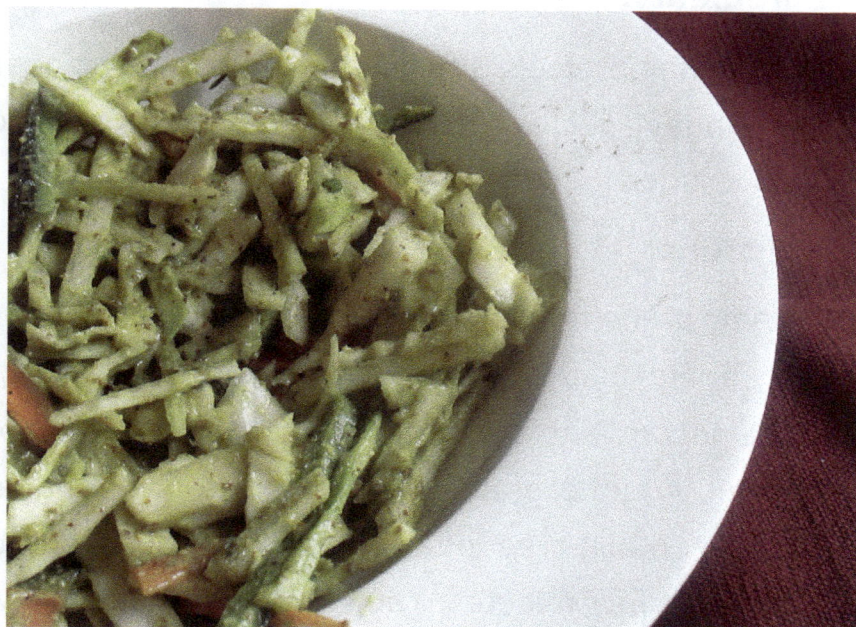

Finger-Licking Appetizer Pretzels

Preparation time: 10 minutes Cooking time: 40 minutes 5 cups.

Ingredients:

3 cups small pretzels 3 tbsp. soy sauce 1 tsp. cinnamon 3 tbsp. agave nectar 2 cups unsalted peanuts or almonds ½ tsp. ginger

Directions:

Begin by preheating the oven to 300 degrees Fahrenheit. Next, bring together the soy sauce, the cinnamon, the agave nectar, and the ginger in a medium-sized bowl. Stir well. Add the pretzels and the nuts and continue to stir. Spread this creation over a baking sheet, and bake them for twenty minutes. You should stir them every five minutes. Next, allow the pretzels to cool, and set them out as a party appetizer. Enjoy!

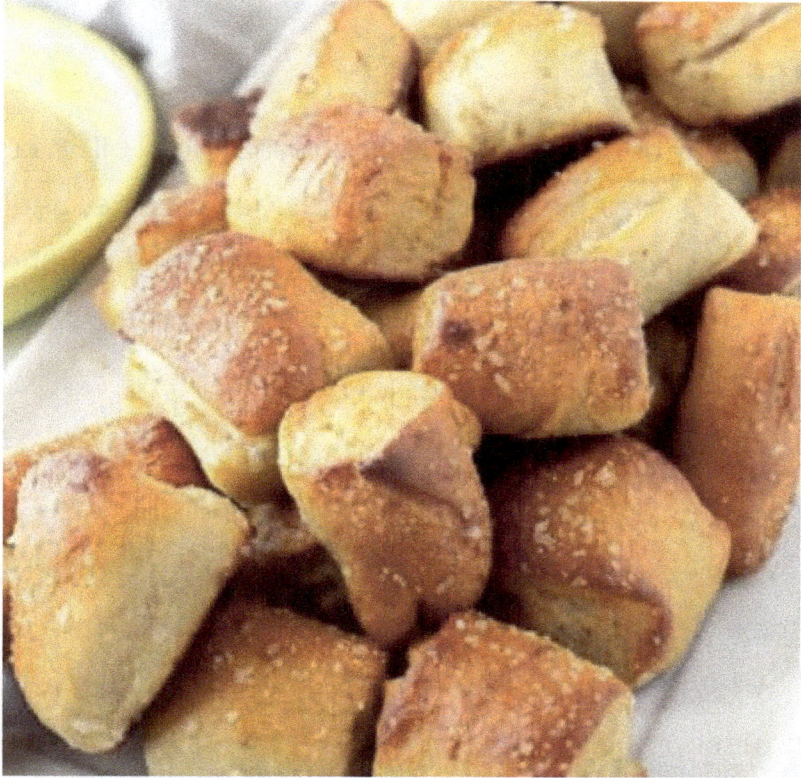

Appetizing Cucumber Salad

Preparation time: 20 minutes Cooking time: 0 minutes Servings: 4

Ingredients:

2 cucumber, peeled 3 tablespoons olive oil 1 cup sour cream 1 tbsp fresh lemon juice 1 garlic clove, peeled and minced 1/3 cup fresh dill leaves, chopped roughly What you'll need from the store cupboard: ½ tsp pepper Salt to taste

Directions:

Slice cucumber into 3 equal lengths. Then slice lengthwise into quarters or smaller to create cucumber sticks. Drain in a colander and set aside. In a medium bowl whisk well the remaining ingredients. Add the drained cucumber into a bowl of dressing and toss well to coat. Serve and enjoy.

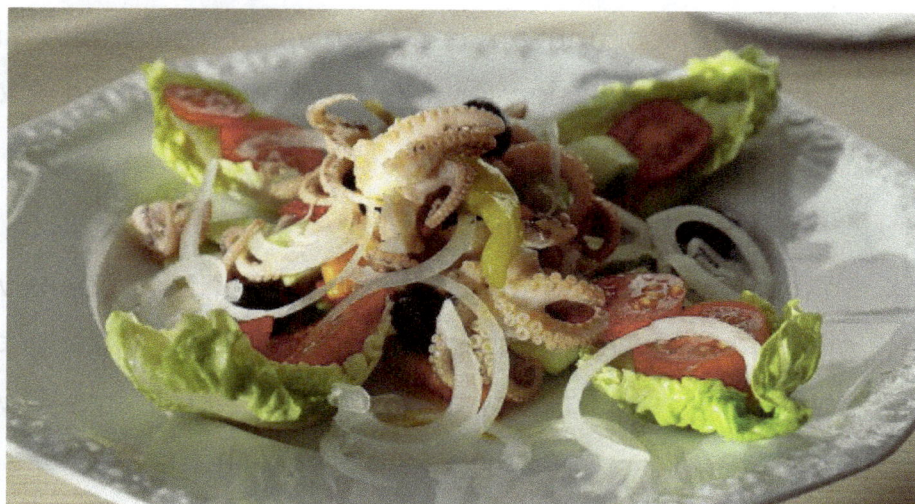

Long Beans Mix

Preparation Time: 10 minutes Cooking Time: 10 minutes Servings:

Ingredients

½ teaspoon coconut aminos 1 tablespoon olive oil A pinch of salt and black pepper 4 garlic cloves, minced 4 long beans, trimmed and sliced

Directions:

In a pan that fits your Air Fryer, combine long beans with oil, aminos, salt, pepper and garlic, toss, introduce in your Air Fryer and cook at 350° F for 10 minutes. Divide between plates and serve as a side dish.

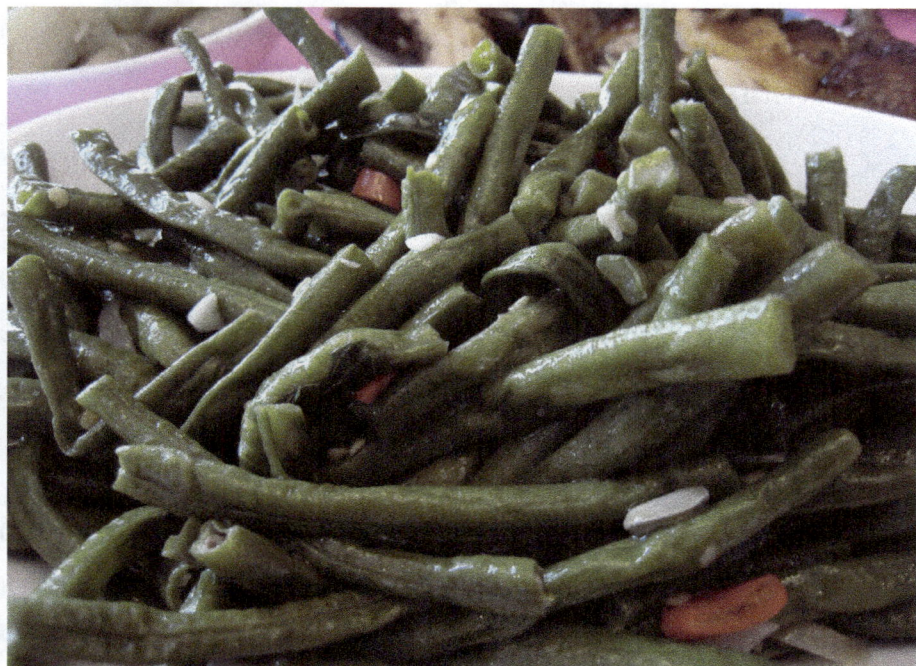

Scalloped Potatoes

Preparation Time: 10 minutes Cooking time: 4 hours Servings: 8

Ingredients:

Cooking spray 2 pounds gold potatoes, halved and sliced 1 yellow onion, cut into medium wedges 10 ounces canned vegan potato cream soup 8 ounces coconut milk 1 cup tofu, crumbled ½ cup veggie stock Salt and black pepper to the taste 1 tablespoons parsley, chopped

Directions:

Coat your slow cooker with cooking spray and arrange half of the potatoes on the bottom. Layer onion wedges, half of the vegan cream soup, coconut milk, tofu, stock, salt and pepper. Add the rest of the potatoes, onion wedges, cream, coconut milk, tofu and stock, cover and cook on High for 4 hours. Sprinkle parsley on top, divide scalloped potatoes between plates and serve as a side dish. Enjoy!

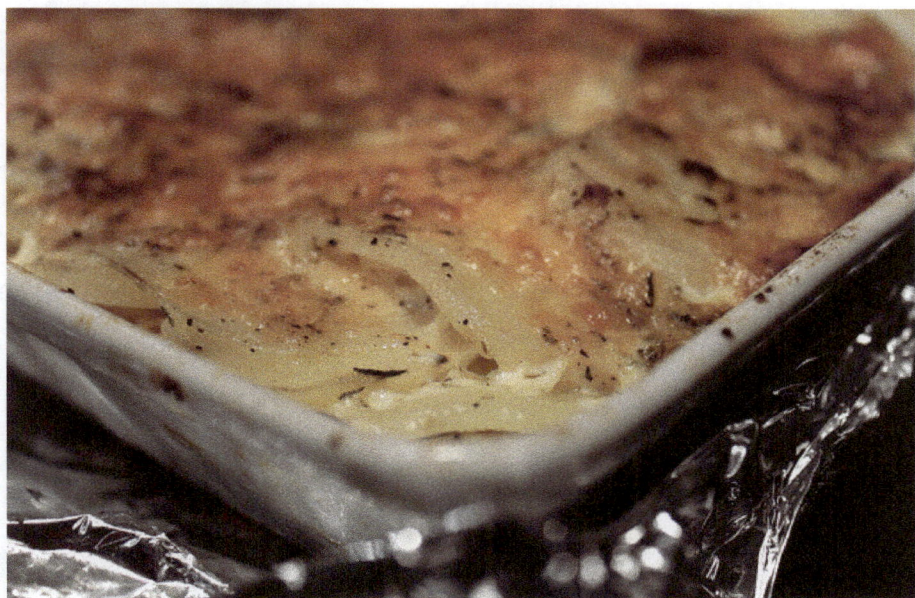

Cauliflower And Broccoli Side Dish

Preparation Time: 10 minutes Cooking time: 3 hours
Servings: 10

Ingredients:

4 cups broccoli florets 4 cups cauliflower florets 14 ounces tomato paste 1 yellow onion, chopped 1 teaspoon thyme, dried Salt and black pepper to the taste ½ cup almonds, sliced

Directions:

In your slow cooker, mix broccoli with cauliflower, tomato paste, onion, thyme, salt and pepper, toss, cover and cook on High for 3 hours. Add almonds, toss, divide between plates and serve as a side dish. Enjoy!

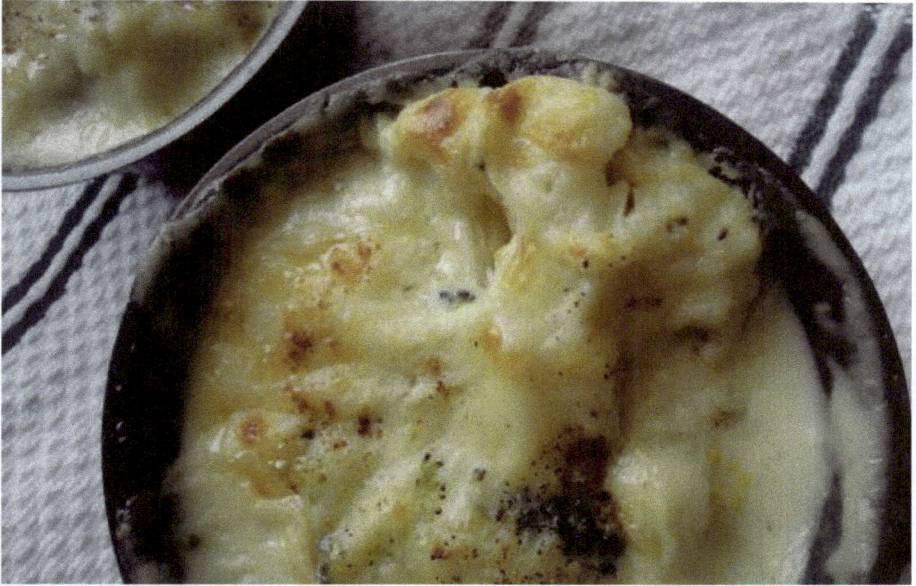

Sun-Dried Tomato Salad And Cider Dressing

Preparation Time: 10 minutes Cooking Time: 10 minutes Serving Yields: 2

Ingredients:

Chopped cucumber - .5 of 1 Sundried tomatoes in the oil – 2 tbsp. Shaved carrots - 3 Thinly sliced red pepper – 1 Sunflower seeds – 1 tsp. Dressing Ingredients: Dijon mustard – 1 tsp. Sunflower oil – 1 tsp. Apple cider vinegar – 1 tsp. Dried oregano - .25 tsp. Dried basil - .25 tsp. White powdered stevia – 1 pinch Herbamare - .125 tsp.

Directions:

Toss all of the veggies into a salad mixing dish along with the sunflower seeds. Whisk the dressing fixings well. Pour the dressing over the tossed salad and serve.

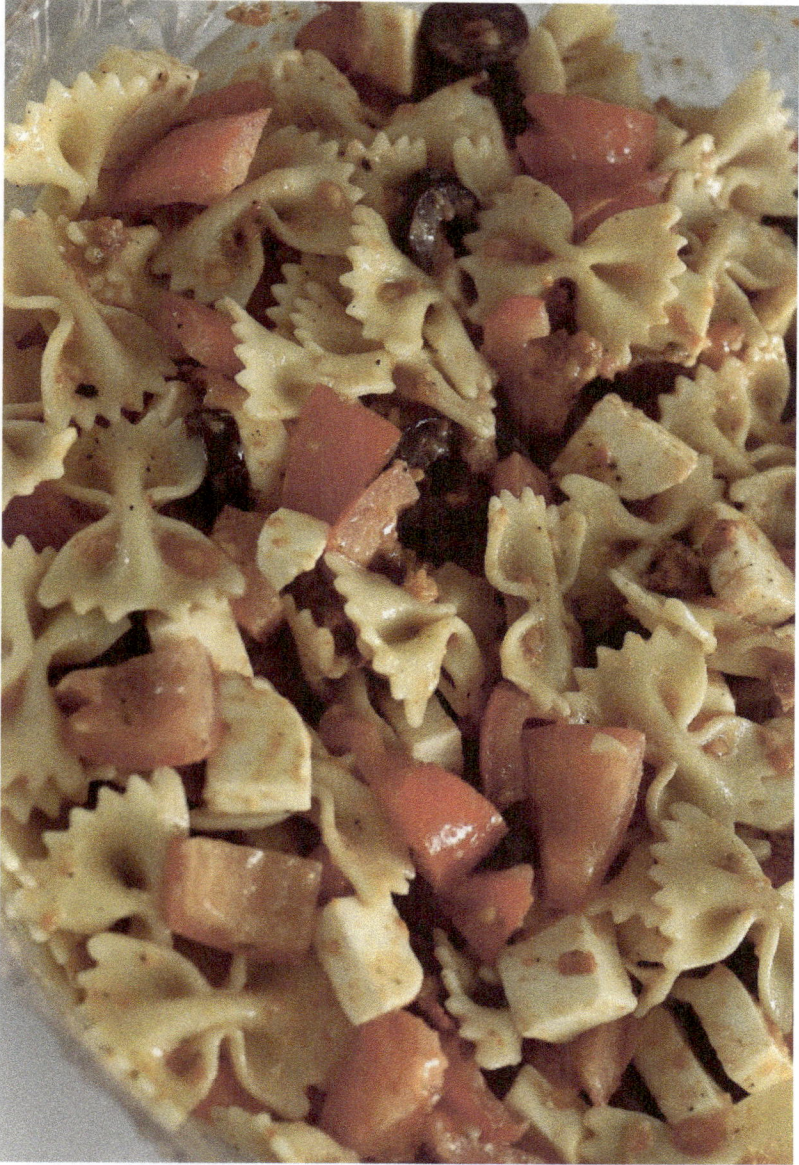

Avocado Pudding

Preparation Time: 10 minutes Serves: 8

Ingredients:

2 ripe avocados, peeled, pitted and cut into pieces 1 tbsp fresh lime juice 14 oz can coconut milk 80 drops of liquid stevia 2 tsp vanilla extract

Directions:

Add all Ingredients into the blender and blend until smooth. Serve and enjoy.

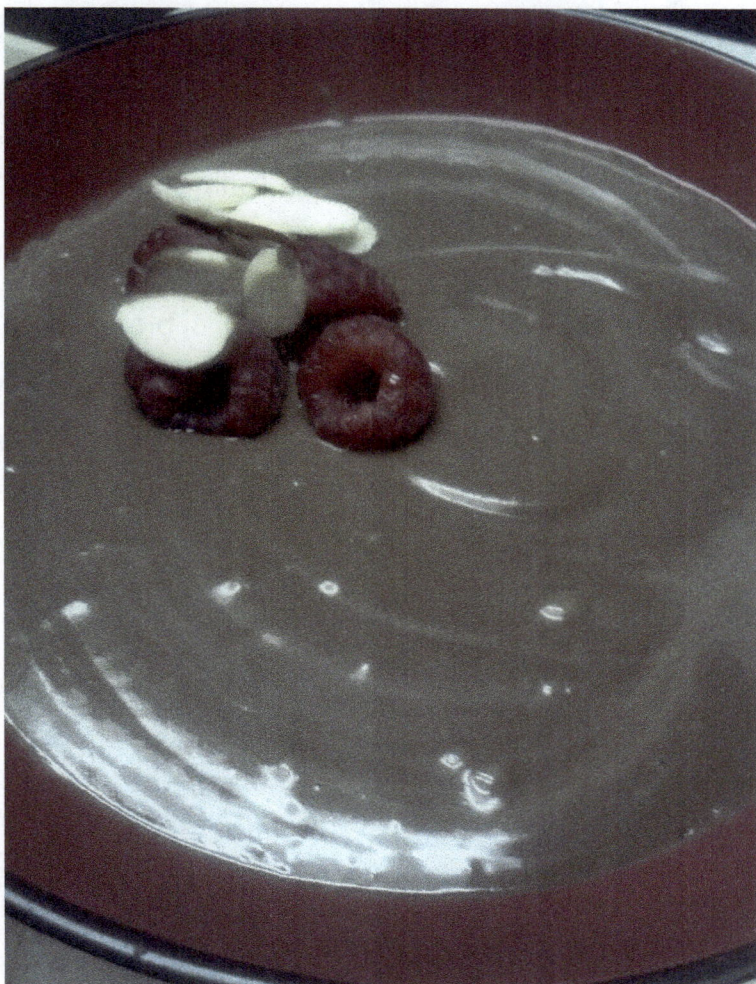

Raspberry Chia Pudding

Preparation Time: 3 hours 10 minutes Serves: 2

Ingredients:

4 tbsp chia seeds 1 cup coconut milk 1/2 cup raspberries

Directions:

Add raspberry and coconut milk in a blender and blend until smooth. Pour mixture into the Mason jar. Add chia seeds in a jar and stir well. Close jar tightly with lid and shake well. Place in refrigerator for 3 hours. Serve chilled and enjoy.

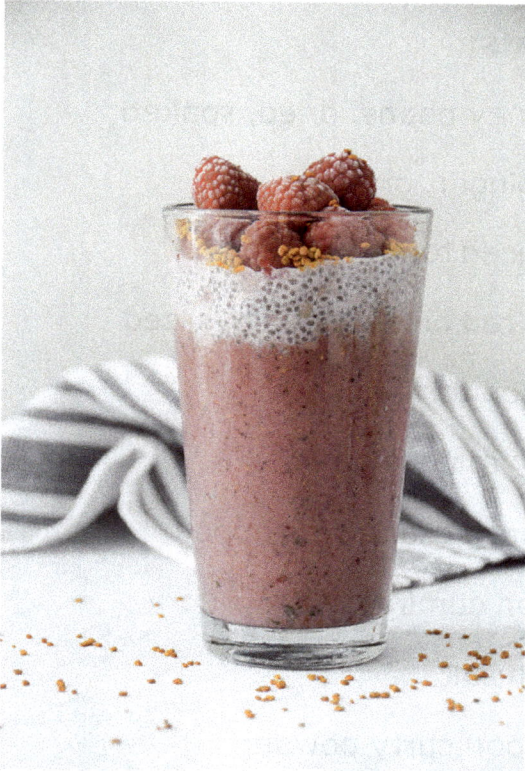

Beans Curry

Preparation time: 10 minutes Cooking time: 8 hours and 10 minutes Servings: 5

Ingredients:

2 cups kidney beans, dried, soaked

1-inch of ginger, grated

1 ½ cup diced tomatoes

1 medium red onion, peeled, sliced

1 tablespoon tomato paste

1 teaspoon minced garlic

1 small bunch cilantro, chopped

½ teaspoon cumin powder

1 teaspoon salt

1 ½ teaspoon curry powder

2 tablespoons olive oil

2 tablespoons lemon juice

Directions:

Place onion in a food processor, add ginger and garlic, and pulse for 1 minute until blended. Take a skillet pan, place it over medium heat, add oil and when hot, add the onion-garlic mixture, and cook for 5 minutes until softened and light brown. Then add tomatoes and tomato paste, stir in ½ teaspoon salt, cumin and curry powder and cook for 5 minutes until cooked. Drain the soaked beans, add them to the slow cooker, add cooked tomato mixture, and remaining ingredients except for cilantro and lemon juice and stir until mixed. Switch on the slow cooker, then shut with lid and cook for 8 hours at high heat setting until tender. When done, transfer 1 cup of beans to the blender, process until creamy, then return it into the slow cooker and stir until mixed. Drizzle with lemon juice, top with cilantro, and serve

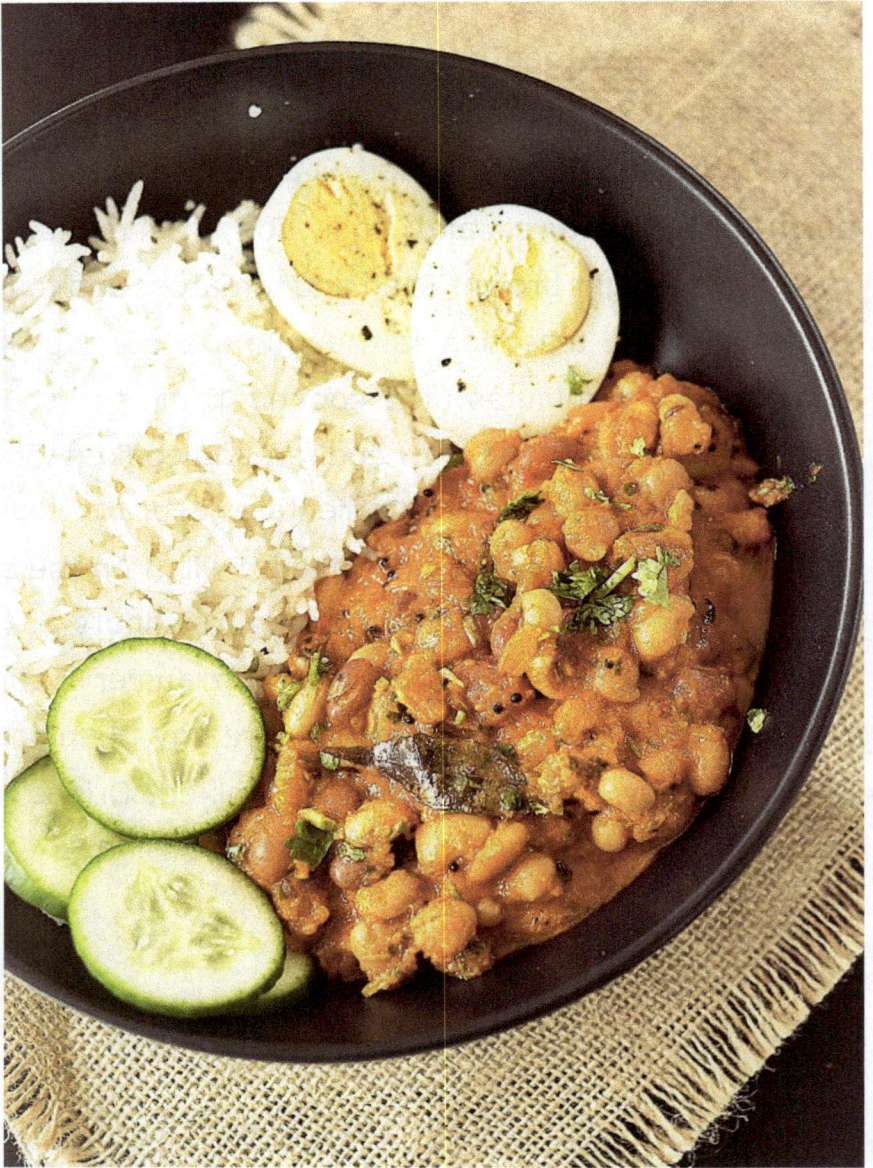

Stuffed Peppers with Kidney Beans

Preparation time: 5 minutes Cooking time: 35 minutes Servings: 4

Ingredients:

3.5 ounces cooked kidney beans 1 big tomato, diced 3.5 ounces sweet corn, canned 2 medium bell peppers, deseeded, halved ½ of medium red onion, peeled, diced 1 teaspoon garlic powder 1/3 teaspoon ground black pepper 2/3 teaspoon salt ½ teaspoon dried basil 3 teaspoons parsley ½ teaspoon dried thyme 3 tablespoons cashew 1 teaspoon olive oil

Directions:

Switch on the oven, then set it to 400 degrees F and let it preheat. Take a large skillet pan, place it over medium heat, add oil and when hot, add onion and cook for 2 minutes until translucent. Add beans, tomatoes, and corn, stir in garlic and cashews and cook for 5 minutes. Stir in salt, black pepper, parsley, basil, and thyme, remove the pan from heat and evenly divide the mixture between bell peppers. Bake the peppers for 25 minutes until tender, then top with parsley and serve.

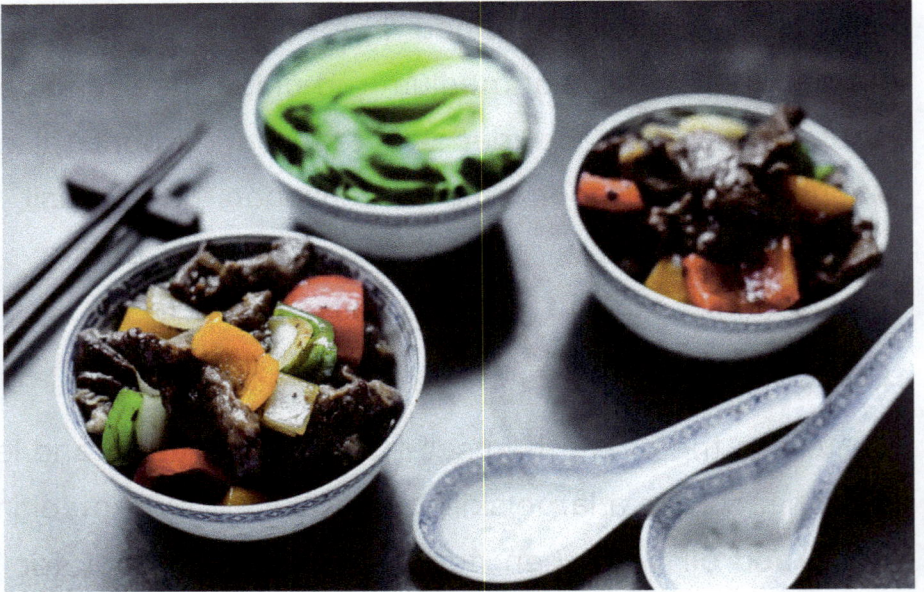

Thai Tofu

Preparation time: 5 minutes Cooking time: 7 minutes Servings: 4

Ingredients:

14 ounces tofu, firm, drained, 3/4 inch cubed 1/3 cup chopped green onion 2 teaspoons grated ginger 3 tablespoons coconut flakes 1 teaspoon soy sauce 1 ½ teaspoon olive oil ¼ cup peanut butter ½ teaspoon sesame oil 1 teaspoon sesame seeds

Directions:

Take a skillet pan, place it over medium-high heat. Reduce heat to medium, add both oils and when hot, add green onions and cook for 1 minute. Then add tofu cubes, cook for 4 minutes and stir in soy sauce halfway. Stir in ginger and peanut butter, stir gently until well incorporated, and then remove the pan from heat. Sprinkle with sesame seeds and serve.

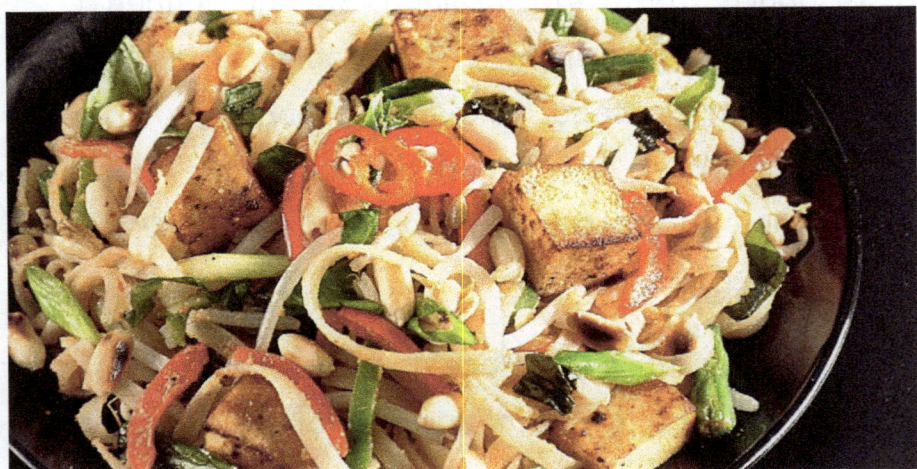

Butternut Squash Linguine

Preparation time: 10 minutes Cooking time: 35 minutes
Servings: 4

Ingredients:

1 medium white onion, peeled, chopped

3 cups diced butternut squash, peeled, deseeded

1 teaspoon minced garlic

½ teaspoon salt

⅛ teaspoon red pepper flakes

¼ teaspoon ground black pepper

1 tablespoon chopped sage

2 tablespoons olive oil

2 cups vegetable broth

12 ounces linguine, whole-grain, cooked

Directions:

Take a large skillet pan, place it over medium heat, add oil and when hot, add sage and cook for 3 minutes until crispy. Transfer sage to a bowl, sprinkle with some salt and set aside until required. Add onion, squash pieces, and garlic into the pan, season with salt, red pepper and black pepper, stir until mixed and cook for 10 minutes. Pour in broth, stir, bring the mixture to boil, then switch heat to medium-low level and simmer for 20 minutes. When done, remove the pan from heat, puree by using an immersion blender until smooth, taste to adjust seasoning and return it into the pan. Heat the pan over medium heat, add cooked pasta, toss until well coated and cook for 2 minutes until hot. Serve straight away.

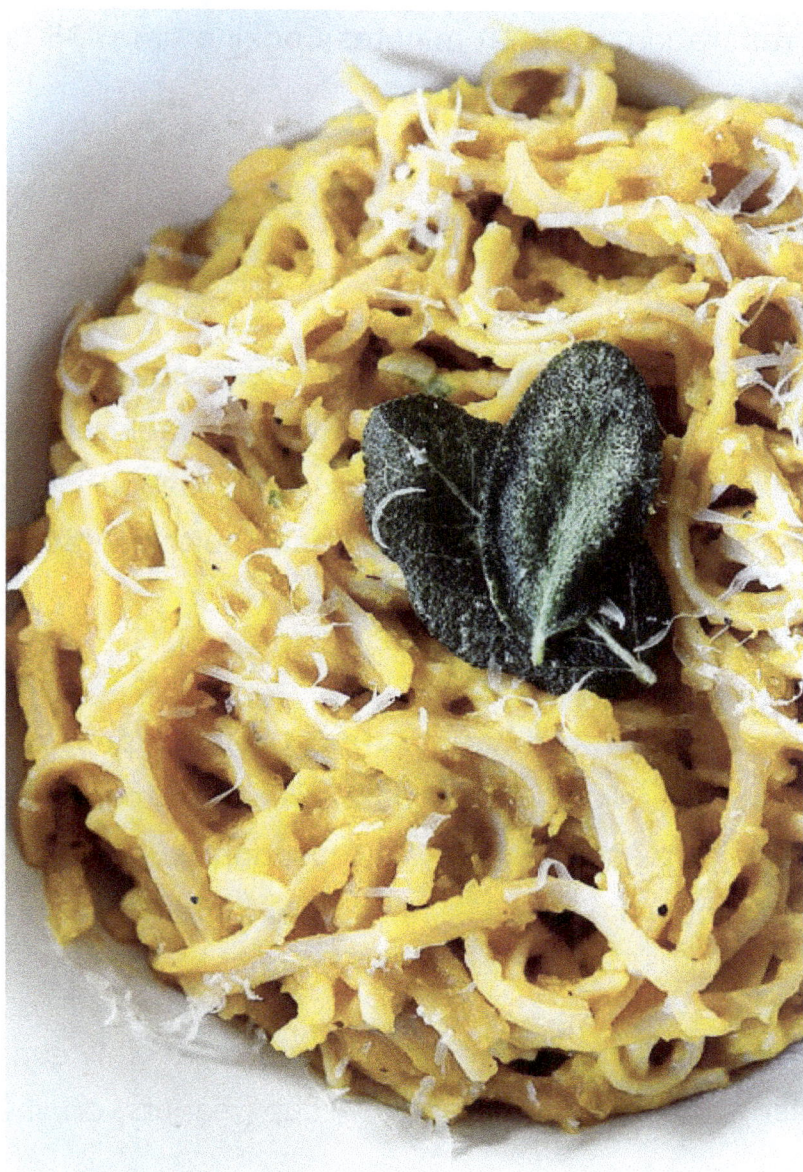

Thai Peanut Sauce over Roasted Sweet Potatoes

Preparation time: 10 minutes Cooking time: 35 minutes
Servings: 4

Ingredients:

For the Thai Peanut Sauce: 1 teaspoon grated ginger 1 teaspoon garlic ¼ cup of soy sauce 3 tablespoons apple cider vinegar ¼ teaspoon red pepper flakes 2 tablespoons honey ½ cup peanut butter 2 tablespoons water

For the Roasted vegetables: 1 red bell pepper, cored, deseeded, sliced into strips 2 sweet potatoes, peeled, 1-inch 1 teaspoon salt ¼ teaspoon cumin powder 2 tablespoons olive oil

For the Garnish: 3 green onions, sliced 1 ¼ cup brown rice, cooked ½ cup cilantro ¼ cup peanuts, crushed

Directions:

Prepare the vegetables and for this, place sweet potatoes on a baking sheet, drizzle with 1 tablespoon oil, season with ½ teaspoon salt and 1/8 teaspoon cumin, toss until mixed and roast for 35 minutes at 425 degrees F, tossing halfway. In the meantime, place bell pepper strips on another baking sheet, drizzle with remaining oil, season with remaining salt, and toss until mixed and roast for 20 minutes at 425 degrees F, tossing halfway. While vegetables are roasting, prepare the sauce and for this, place all its ingredients in a bowl and whisk until combined. Distribute rice between four bowls, top with roasted vegetables, drizzle with sauce, garnish with peanuts, cilantro, and green onions, and serve.

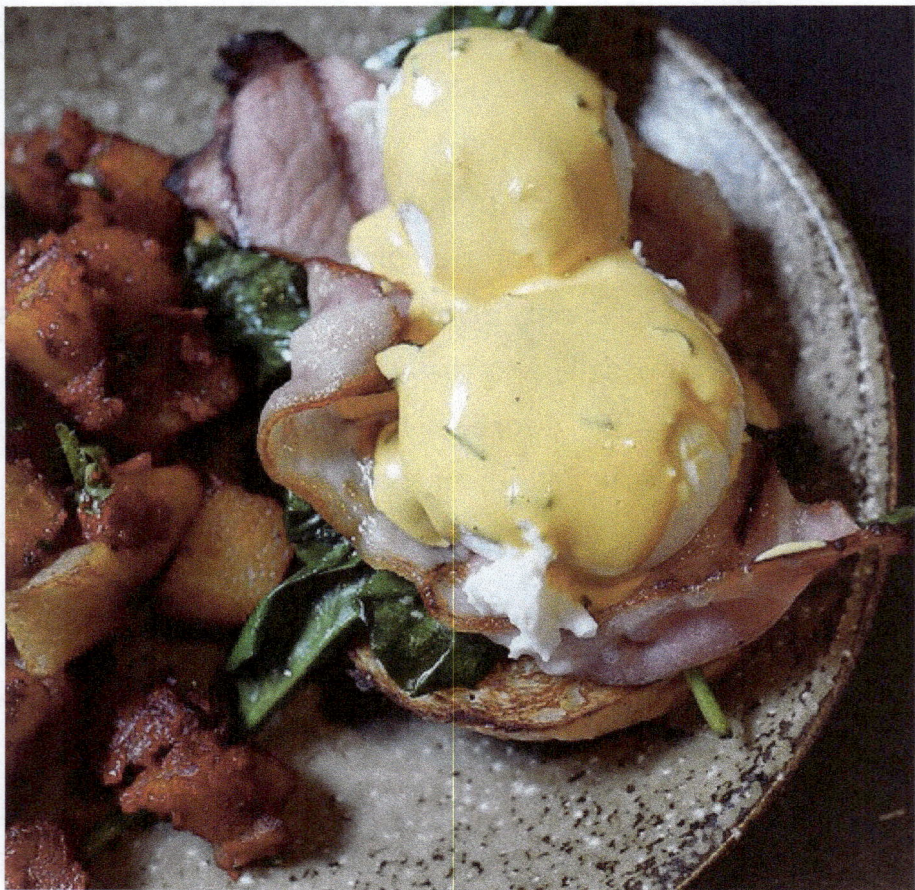

www.ingramcontent.com/pod-product-compliance
Lightning Source LLC
Chambersburg PA
CBHW050755030426
42336CB00012B/1834